Dairy-Free Cookbook for Beginners

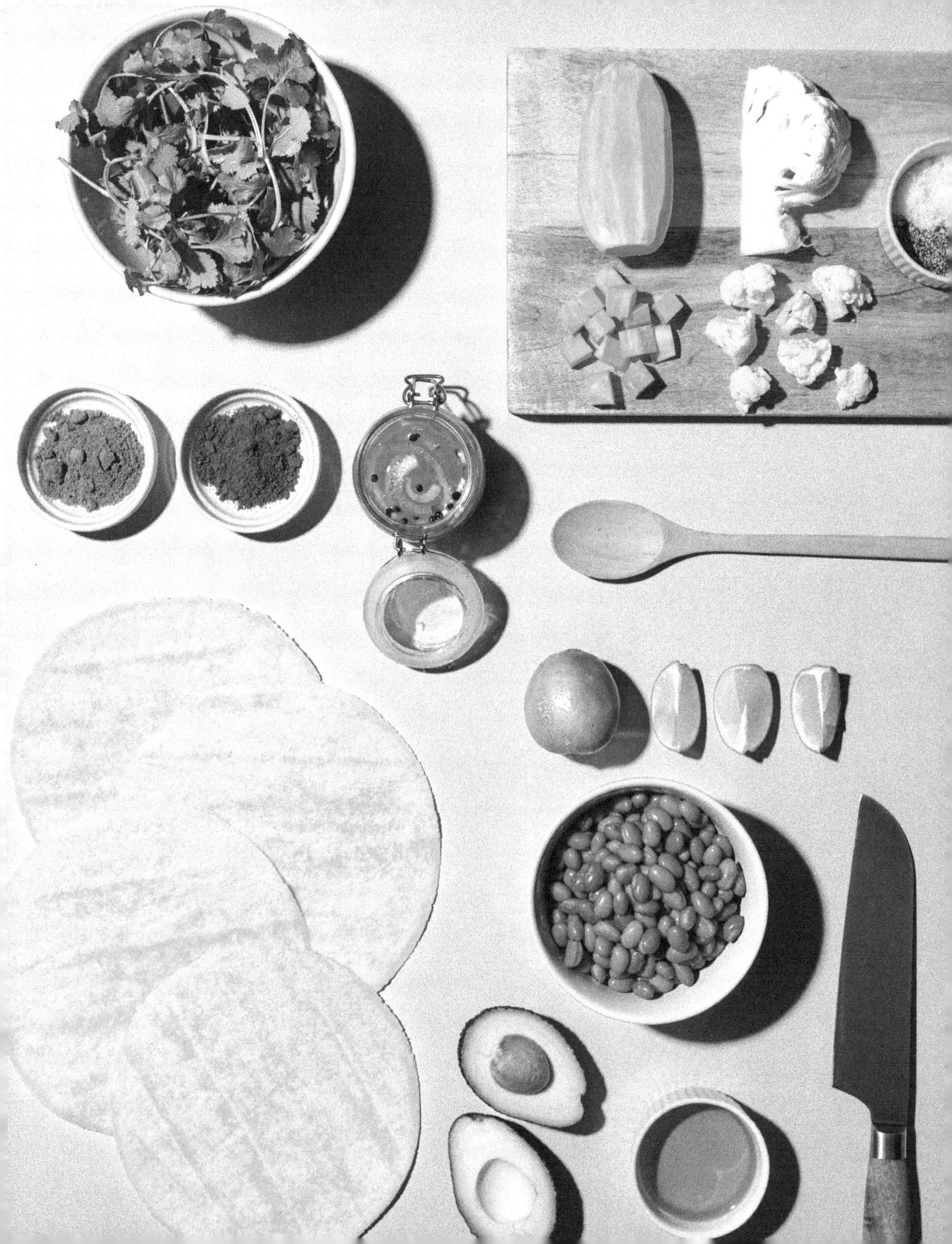

# DAIRY-FREE COOKBOOK for Beginners

## 101 Simple, Satisfying Recipes

Chrissy Carroll, MPH, RD

Photography by Darren Muir

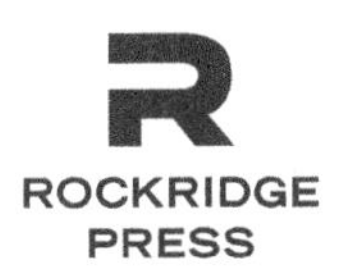

For general information on our other products and services or to obtain technical support, please contact our Customer Care Department within the United States at (866) 744-2665, or outside the United States at (510) 253-0500.

Rockridge Press publishes its books in a variety of electronic and print formats. Some content that appears in print may not be available in electronic books, and vice versa.



Interior and Cover Designer: Darren Samuel
Art Producer: Sue Bischofberger
Editor: Anna Pulley
Production Manager: Michael Kay
Production Editor: Sigi Nacson



ISBN: Print 978-1-64739-012-9 | Ebook 978-1-64739-013-6

R0

For Devon, my crazy-haired kiddo—I'm forever grateful for your enthusiasm and kind heart.

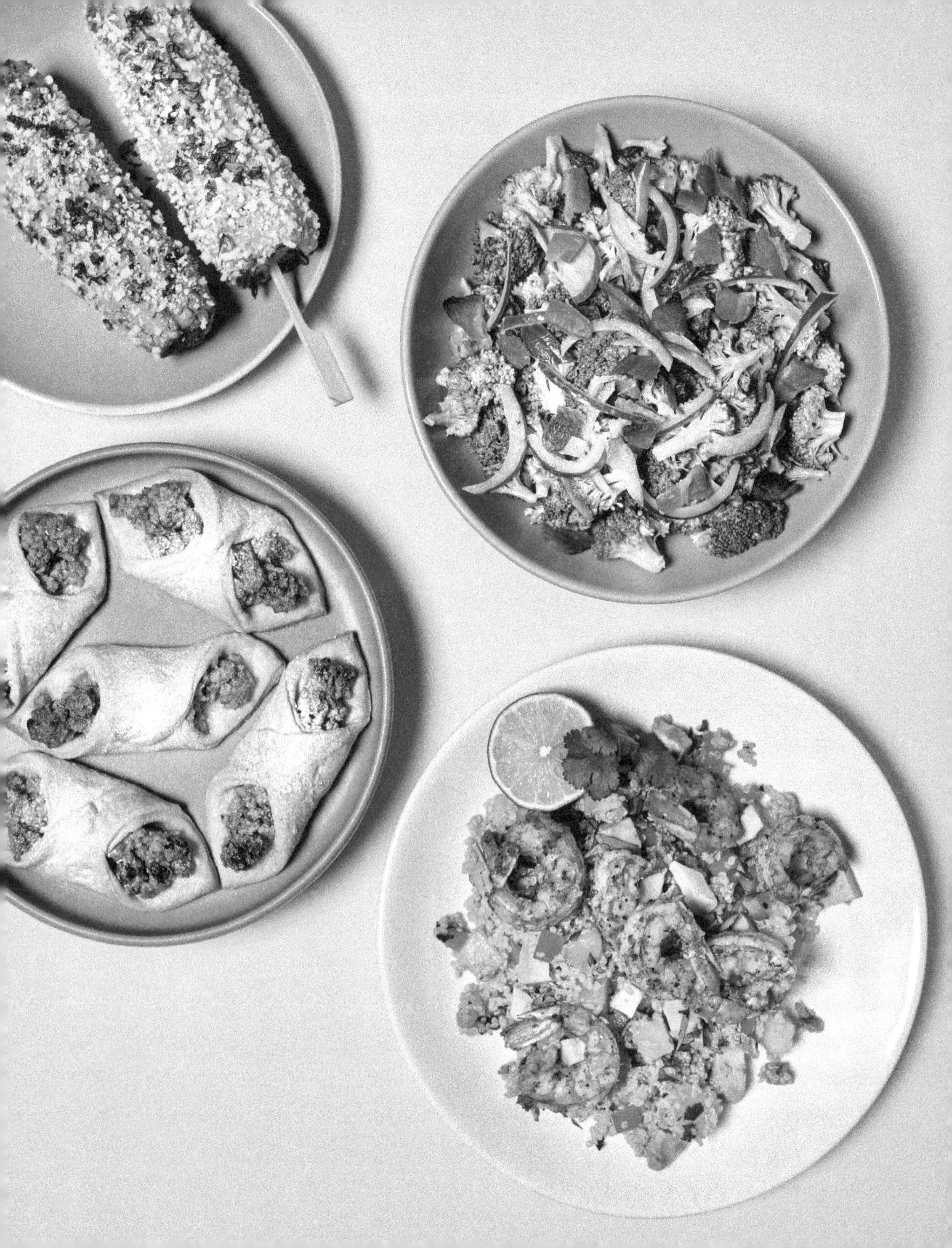

# CONTENTS

# INTRODUCTION

Welcome to the world of dairy-free cooking! Whether you're excited to get started or completely overwhelmed by the prospect of leaving your dairy favorites behind, I look forward to guiding you on this journey and showing you how to make a dairy-free lifestyle work for you.

My personal experience with dairy-free eating began just a few weeks after my son was born, when he was diagnosed with food protein–induced allergic proctocolitis. In layperson's terms, he couldn't digest certain food proteins—specifically dairy, soy, and eggs. Since I was nursing at the time, I was thrust into overhauling my own diet in order to keep him healthy.

Even as a registered dietitian, I found it overwhelming to try to balance this new way of eating while simultaneously learning to parent a newborn. I found it especially challenging to think through meal ideas and read every label. Although I knew dishes like grilled chicken and steamed broccoli were "safe," I wanted recipes that were hearty and indulgent, too.

I quickly realized many other parents—many of whom didn't have the nutrition background and culinary knowledge I did—were struggling with the same thing. That realization became my catalyst to embrace dairy-free cooking, learn how to re-create classic favorites, make soul-satisfying meals, and create rich desserts, all without dairy. After many years of recipe experiments and testing, I've amassed a treasure trove of self-created recipes that you'll find in this cookbook and on my website, Dairy Free for Baby.

Let's talk about why you're here. You may be struggling with a similar situation with your own child, or have been diagnosed with an allergy or intolerance yourself. Perhaps you're choosing a dairy-free lifestyle for other reasons, like digestive health or ethical beliefs. No matter the reason, here you'll find a clear, simple path to learn about and start a dairy-free diet.

Don't let the word "diet" worry you. Despite the fact that I may refer to this as a "diet," it's really a lifestyle change. Diets sometimes imply deprivation, and you won't feel anything close to that with these recipes. I'm here to show you how you can still enjoy just about any of your favorite meals with easy swaps and modifications that you will come to feel quite at home with.

We'll talk about the tools, tips, and key ingredients you'll want to know about in order to optimize your new way of living. And then we'll dive into the recipes—101 easy recipes for everything from sauces to main dishes to holiday treats. Before you know it, you'll be cooking up tasty dairy-free meals that satisfy you, your family, and your dinner guests alike. Ready to dive in? Grab your plant-based milk and vegan butter, and let's get started!

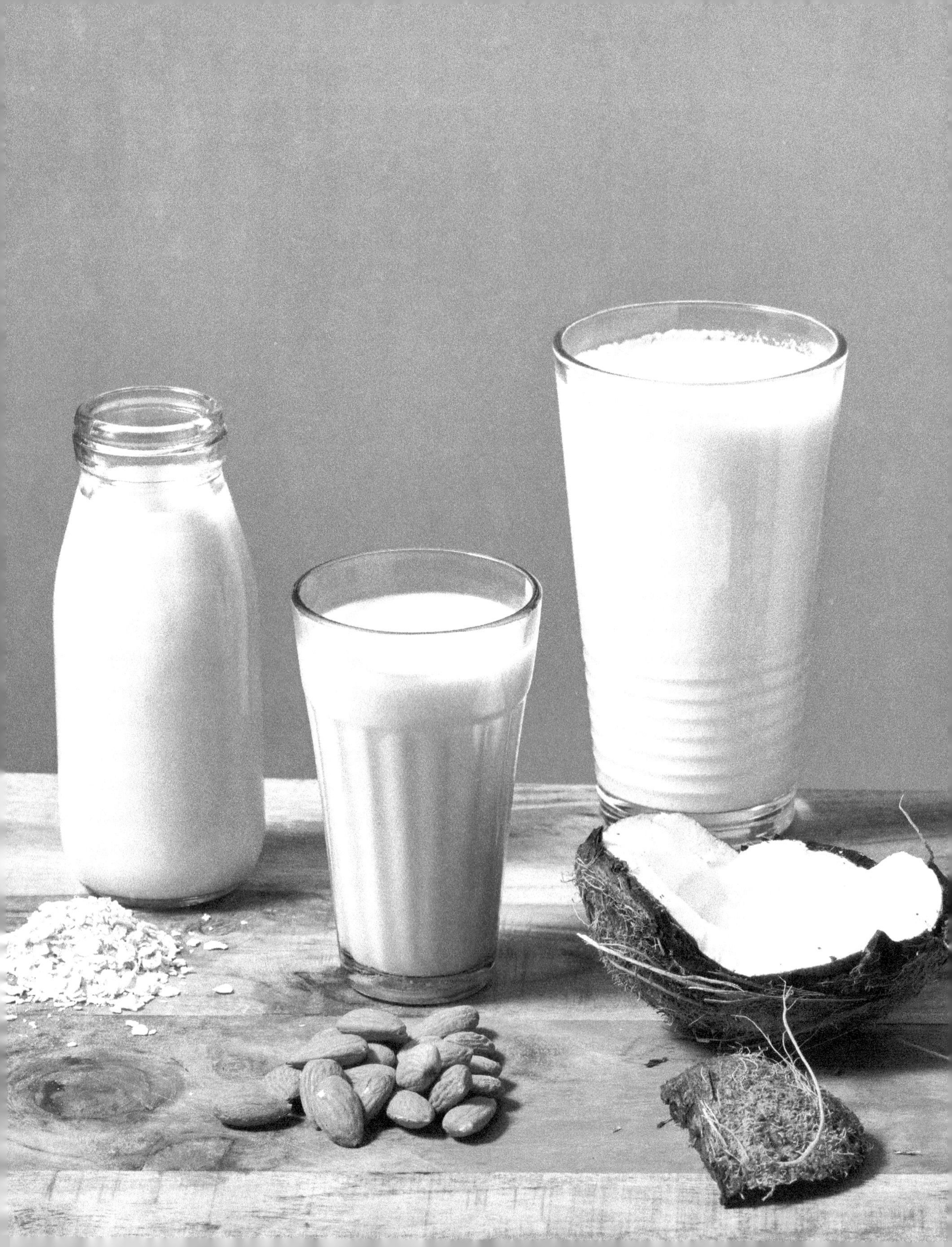

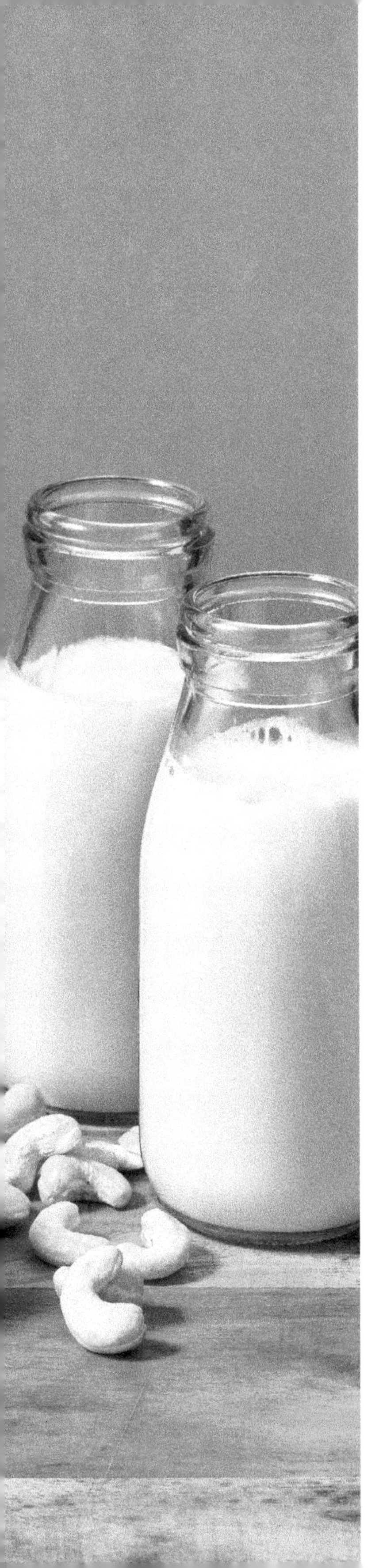

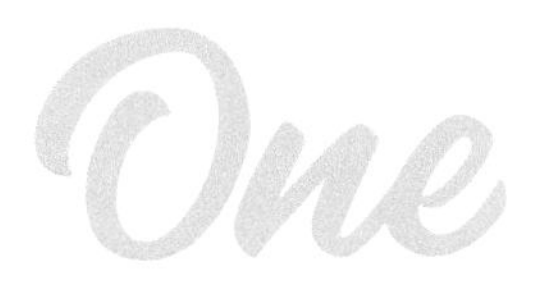

# Dairy-Free 101

Change can be intimidating—and that's especially true when you're embarking on a new way of eating. But with a little planning, preparation, and creativity, you'll find that dairy-free living can be both doable and delicious. You'll soon be able to whip up anything from a nutritious dinner to a decadent dessert, all while meeting your dietary needs.

Throughout this chapter, you'll find helpful tips on the benefits of dairy-free eating, label-reading, plant-based substitutes, and more.

## The Benefits of Dairy-Free Eating

If you think you're making a sacrifice by giving up dairy, you're not alone. Forgoing your favorite cheese or ice cream can feel like a punishment! But soon enough, these changes will become second nature. Not only will you forget about what you're giving up, but you'll also realize everything you're *gaining*, such as exciting, new go-to favorites, and, of course, a healthier way of life.

I don't believe dairy is inherently unhealthy—but it may be the wrong choice for *your* body depending on health concerns or ethical beliefs. You can expect to reap several benefits on this new diet, some that may be specific to medical concerns and others that are universal:

**Prevents allergic reactions.** It can be quite scary to learn you (or your nursing baby) have a food allergy. Allergies involve an immune system attack on a particular protein—in this case, the protein in milk products. Because allergies can progress in severity, it's essential to eliminate all dairy products from your diet. By doing so, you're keeping your body safe and preventing uncomfortable, unhealthy, and even life-threatening reactions.

**Eliminates lactose intolerance symptoms.** Unlike an allergy where protein in milk is a concern, lactose intolerance is the inability to fully digest the sugar in milk. It's less severe, but can still have some pretty uncomfortable side effects, such as diarrhea, bloating, or gas. Switching to low-lactose products or ditching dairy altogether can help you feel better and eliminate these symptoms.

**Clears skin.** Research suggests dairy may be associated with acne in adolescents and young adults. A study in the journal *Nutrients* concluded that dairy products were associated with increased risk of acne among those from ages 7 to 30. Additionally, infants and young children with dairy allergies may have eczema that's exacerbated by eating dairy products. Removing dairy from the diet may help clear up the skin.

**Indirectly promotes weight loss.** Dairy itself has not been proven to contribute to excess weight gain or obesity. However, when following a dairy-free diet, you'll need to eliminate some of the dairy-containing processed foods you used to eat. You'll probably also find yourself cooking more at home, rather than eating out or grabbing on-the-go convenience foods. These choices may indirectly help you lose weight.

**Improves symptoms of digestive disorders.** Dairy products may trigger symptoms in certain digestive disorders. For example, high-fat dairy products may increase the risk of diarrhea among patients with irritable bowel syndrome. Similarly, some digestive disorders can be exacerbated by a group of carbohydrates known as FODMAPs. Lactose, the sugar found in milk, is one type of FODMAP, which may be related to digestive symptoms in some people. Although not all dairy products contain high levels of fat or lactose, you may choose to eliminate all dairy to see how the body reacts.

**Aligns with your ethical beliefs.** You may choose to eliminate dairy because of ethical beliefs surrounding animal food products or agricultural sustainability. By choosing a dairy-free lifestyle, you're able to assert your beliefs in an actionable way that makes you feel good.

No matter your reason for going dairy-free, this process will help you better connect with your body. You'll refine your skills in the kitchen, learn more about label-reading and associated terms, and make changes that can positively impact your health.

## What Is a Dairy-Free Diet?

A dairy-free diet eliminates all forms of dairy, which includes both whole foods and individual ingredients. When you first start this diet, you may be surprised to see how many processed foods contain dairy as an ingredient!

You'll want to hone your label-reading skills to assess if a food is truly dairy-free. Use the following lists to assist you. Since milk is one of the top eight allergens (along with eggs, fish, shellfish, peanuts, wheat, soybeans, and tree nuts), it must be declared on most food labels. It can be listed in plain language in the ingredients or in a "contains: milk" statement.

### FOODS THAT DEFINITELY HAVE DAIRY

You'll want to avoid these obvious sources of dairy:

- Butter (and most forms of this word, such as butter solids and butterfat)
- Cheese
- Cottage cheese
- Cream
- Ghee
- Half-and-half
- Ice cream
- Kefir
- Milk (and most forms of this word, such as buttermilk and fat-free milk powder)
- Pudding
- Ricotta
- Sour cream
- Whipped cream
- Yogurt (including regular, Greek, quark, and skyr)

### FOODS THAT MAY HAVE DAIRY

Skipping the milk and cheese is simple, but there are other surprising foods that sometimes contain dairy. Always check the ingredients on these foods, as some brands will be safe and others will not:

- Bread
- Caramel flavoring
- Chocolate (even dark)
- Crackers
- Flavored potato chips
- Hot dogs
- Imitation crab
- Margarine

- Mashed potatoes
- "Nondairy" foods (like creamer or ice cream labeled as "nondairy")
- Nougat
- Salad dressings
- Sausages
- Sherbet
- Tuna in cans or pouches

## HIDDEN FORMS OF DAIRY IN INGREDIENT LISTS

Dairy can be listed in many ways on a label's ingredient list. If it's not listed in plain language, the manufacturer should make it clear that the product contains milk. However, be aware of these sneaky words, which indicate dairy:

- **Casein and caseinates:** Casein is one of the two main proteins found in milk. Avoid products that include casein or any type of caseinate (ammonium caseinate, sodium caseinate, etc.).
- **Lactose and other "lact" words:** Lactose is the sugar found in milk. Other "lact" words can indicate dairy-derived ingredients as well (with a few exceptions found in the next section). Avoid ingredients like lactalbumin, lactalbumin phosphate, lactoglobulin, lactate solids, and lactulose.
- **Nisin preparation:** This food preservative is typically derived from milk, though there are nondairy nisin preparations on the market, too.
- **Simplesse:** This dairy- and egg-based product is used in low-calorie/low-fat foods to achieve a certain texture and mouthfeel.
- **Recaldent:** Although Recaldent isn't as common as it used to be, some chewing gums use this milk-based product as a functional ingredient for delivering calcium and phosphate to teeth.
- **Whey:** Whey is the second type of protein found in dairy, and all forms of it should be avoided.

## SURPRISINGLY DAIRY-FREE INGREDIENTS/FOODS

Enjoy these ingredients without worry—although they sound like they have dairy (and you should double-check labels), they're generally safe:

- Cocoa butter
- Cocoa powder (unsweetened)
- Coconut butter (sometimes called coconut manna)
- Coconut cream
- Cream of tartar
- Fruit butters
- Lactic acid (however, lactic acid starter culture may contain dairy)
- Nut butters
- Sodium or calcium lactate

## INFANT DAIRY ALLERGIES

Finding out your little one has a dairy allergy can be scary! Several different conditions are lumped under this category, but no matter which condition your baby has, the treatment remains the same if dairy is the culprit: eliminate dairy from the diet. For infants, that will either mean changing your own diet to continue nursing, or introducing a formula that they can tolerate.

If choosing formula, your doctor may recommend an extensively hydrolyzed formula (EHF) or an elemental formula. In an EHF, the milk proteins are broken down into very small pieces that are tolerated by some babies with milk allergies. In an elemental formula, the base is made up of amino acids rather than full proteins, with no intact milk proteins at all.

As your child transitions to table food, continue serving them dairy-free dishes. This cookbook contains many kid-friendly recipes, including Belgian Waffles (page 49) and Mango Avocado Salad (page 59).

The good news is that many children outgrow these allergies and intolerances. Always check with your doctor before reintroducing foods, as your child may need to be tested in-office depending on their specific condition.

# Essential Substitutions

For every common dairy staple, there's a delicious alternative that will fit your new diet.

### INSTEAD OF BUTTER: *TRY COOKING OILS OR VEGAN BUTTER.*

Oils are an easy swap for butter when you're sautéing vegetables or panfrying meat. Olive oil is a clear winner to keep in your kitchen, since you can use this versatile oil for anything from roasting vegetables to creating homemade salad dressings. I also keep canola oil, peanut oil, and avocado oil stocked for frying, as all have fairly high smoke points. Coconut oil is great for sautéing and baking, though some people don't like the slight coconut flavor it imparts.

You'll also want to keep vegan butter on hand. This product creates the right flavor and texture in certain baked goods and desserts (like biscuits or a buttercream frosting).

### INSTEAD OF SEMI-HARD CHEESE: *TRY A DAIRY-FREE CHEESE.*

Ten years ago, you'd be lucky to find even one dairy-free cheese in the store. Today, you'll find many brands made with different bases, from soy to nuts. Experiment with a few to find one that tastes great and works in your recipes. Try them sprinkled on top of your pizza or mixed into a casserole.

### INSTEAD OF PARMESAN: *TRY NUTRITIONAL YEAST.*

Nutritional yeast is made from a strain of yeast that's grown and then processed with heat to deactivate it. Although it sounds a little strange, it adds a wonderful cheesy, savory flavor to dishes. Buy it in dried powder form or flakes and use it to make your own homemade Dairy-Free Parmesan (page 36).

### INSTEAD OF CREAMER: *TRY ALMOND OR COCONUT CREAMER.*

If you're a coffee drinker, stock up on almond- or coconut-based creamers for your cup of joe. Even products advertised as "nondairy" creamers sometimes still contain milk derivatives, so be sure to check the labels.

### INSTEAD OF YOGURT: *TRY DAIRY-FREE YOGURT.*

You can find yogurt made from almond milk, oat milk, and coconut milk. All three are good for snacking, making a breakfast parfait, or baking.

### INSTEAD OF CREAM CHEESE: *TRY CASHEW CHEESE.*

You can make an easy cashew-based cream cheese on your own, like Scallion Cream Cheese (page 35), which packs in a ton of flavor for your bagels. Or stock up on dairy-free cream cheese (often tofu-based) at the grocery store.

### INSTEAD OF FROZEN WHIPPED TOPPING: *TRY COCONUT WHIP.*

If you love strawberry shortcake loaded up with frozen whipped topping, you'll want to try the frozen coconut whips that are now available. These have a delicious flavor and are perfect for fruit desserts.

## Mooove Over Dairy Milk: Types of Plant-Based Milks

A wide variety of plant-based milks means you've got access to the right option for any recipe. You can find unsweetened varieties, which often have less sugar than traditional dairy milk, as well as sweetened varieties for those who prefer a boost of flavor.

Most plant-based milks are fortified with vitamins and minerals, like calcium and vitamin D, to provide amounts comparable to dairy milk. However, not all brands are fortified, so check the nutrition facts if you're relying on milk for those vitamins and minerals.

In fact, there are so many options, you may not know where to start. Here are the details on a few plant-based milks to consider trying:

- **Soy milk:** The texture and nutrition profile of soy milk are similar to dairy milk, and the protein content is higher than that of many alternatives.
- **Pea protein milk:** For those looking to avoid both dairy and soy, pea protein milk is another high-protein choice. You can use it in most applications where you'd use dairy milk.

- **Almond milk:** Unsweetened is perfect for savory dishes, whereas the sweetened varieties work well in baked desserts and sweet breakfasts, or poured over cereal.
- **Coconut milk/cream:** Canned coconut milk has a high fat content, so it works well in recipes that call for cream, like soups and curries.
- **Oat milk:** This is naturally sweeter than most other milk alternatives. It works well in baked goods and sweet breakfast recipes, or poured over cereal.
- **Cashew milk:** This has a creamy, slightly nutty flavor. It tastes great in sauces, soups, and smoothies.

You can make many of these plant-based milks at home, as you'll see in chapter 3; however, don't hesitate to buy them at the store if that's easier.

## Tips for Eating Out

Although eating out might feel challenging, it can still be done on a dairy-free diet. Consider these tips:

- **Look for allergy-friendly restaurants.** They'll be more familiar with the ingredients in their menu items, as well as protocols to prevent cross-contamination. (See the Resources section for more on this.) Local non-chain restaurants are happy to accommodate requests to make dishes dairy-free or suggest those that are already dairy-free.
- **Find vegan options.** Vegan restaurants (and vegan dishes) are an excellent option for dairy-free meals, as all vegan food is dairy-free.
- **Visit restaurant websites.** When visiting a restaurant, especially a chain restaurant, see if allergen information is available online, which allows you to find menu options that do not contain dairy. When you arrive, double-check that your choices are dairy-free by confirming with a manager or the chef, just in case the online resources are outdated.

For severe allergies, keep in mind that cross-contamination can be a concern (such as dairy-containing foods cooked in the same fryers or handled with the same gloves).

- **Choose cuisines wisely.** Try cuisines that are naturally low in dairy ingredients. For example, Thai food and sushi are generally good choices for finding dairy-free options. Be sure to always ask about ingredients, though.

## Frequently Asked Questions about Going Dairy-Free

When starting this journey, you're bound to have questions. There is no such thing as a dumb question; if you're curious about something, odds are that many other people want those answers, too!

Here are some of the top Q&As of dairy-free living. If you have additional concerns, ask a medical professional or a dietitian for personalized guidance.

Q: Can I do this? Can I really live without cheese and butter?

A: You've got this! Although it may seem tough at first, a little self-education can arm you with the knowledge to make dairy-free eating feel like second nature. With so many product alternatives on the market these days, you'll be surprised at how you can make just about any meal dairy-free.

Q: Can I eat eggs?

A: Yes! Since eggs come from chickens rather than cows, they contain no milk protein and are completely acceptable on a dairy-free diet.

Q: How do I get enough calcium?

A: Adults generally need 1,000 mg of calcium each day. Calcium is found in fortified plant-based milks, fortified orange juice, canned fish with bones (like sardines), tofu, and certain leafy greens. If you're worried about meeting your calcium needs, you can also take a calcium supplement.

**Q:** What about parties and holidays? How do I handle those?

**A:** BYOD! By bringing your own dairy-free dishes to share at these events, you know you'll have something delicious to eat. If you're going to a dinner party, it's okay to tell the host ahead of time that you don't eat dairy. Hosting events yourself is another way to be sure the menu works for you!

**Q:** Can dairy be hidden under "natural flavors" on an ingredients label?

**A:** Natural flavors can, in fact, contain dairy; however, this cannot be hidden. Under labeling laws, dairy must be clearly specified in the ingredients or in an allergen statement.

**Q:** Do foods with dairy need to have a "contains: milk" statement?

**A:** One common misconception with labeling is that a food must have a "contains" statement, but this is not the case. As long as dairy is listed in the ingredients in words you understand (milk, cheese, etc.), the manufacturer does not have to use a "contains" statement.

**Q:** What does "may contain milk" mean on a food label?

**A:** This is a voluntary warning for cross-contamination. The product may be manufactured on shared equipment lines as another product that contains dairy. If you have a severe allergy, your doctor may recommend you avoid products with this warning. If you have a mild intolerance or are going dairy-free for other reasons, though, you don't have to worry about this warning.

**Q:** Are there foods that don't have to adhere to allergy labeling laws?

**A:** Yes. The FDA regulates most packaged foods, but they do not cover meat and poultry products, alcoholic beverages, restaurant foods, or anything from a place where a person can buy food to go (like a bakery or food truck). Some of these may contain dairy.

**Q:** What if I have other allergies, too?

**A:** Handling multiple allergies can feel overwhelming, but over time you'll learn what works for you. Although this cookbook is focused exclusively on dairy-free eating, I've included notations for those dishes that are also soy-free, egg-free, nut-free, or gluten-free. With a little creativity, most recipes can be modified with substitutions to fit a variety of allergy concerns.

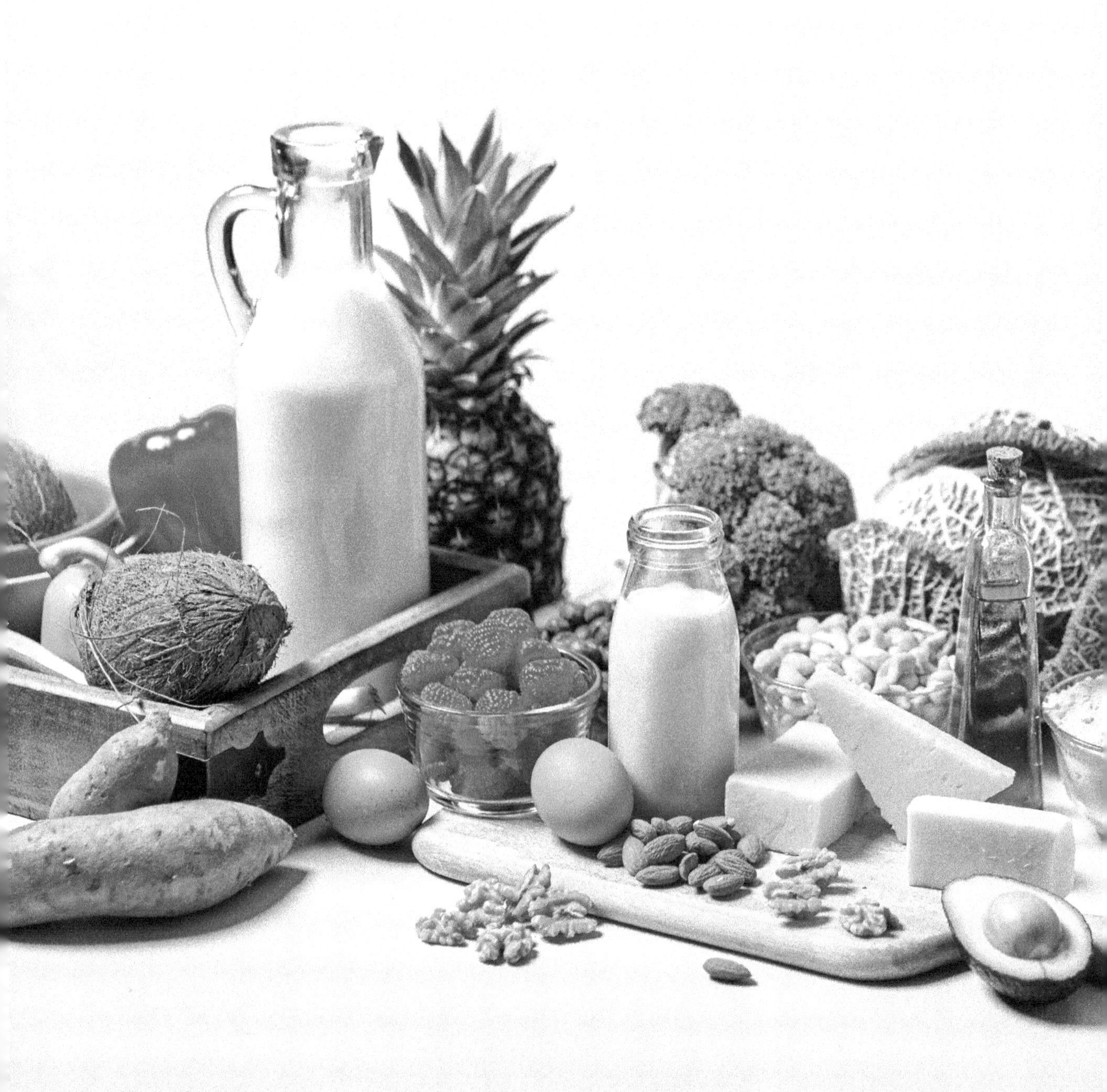

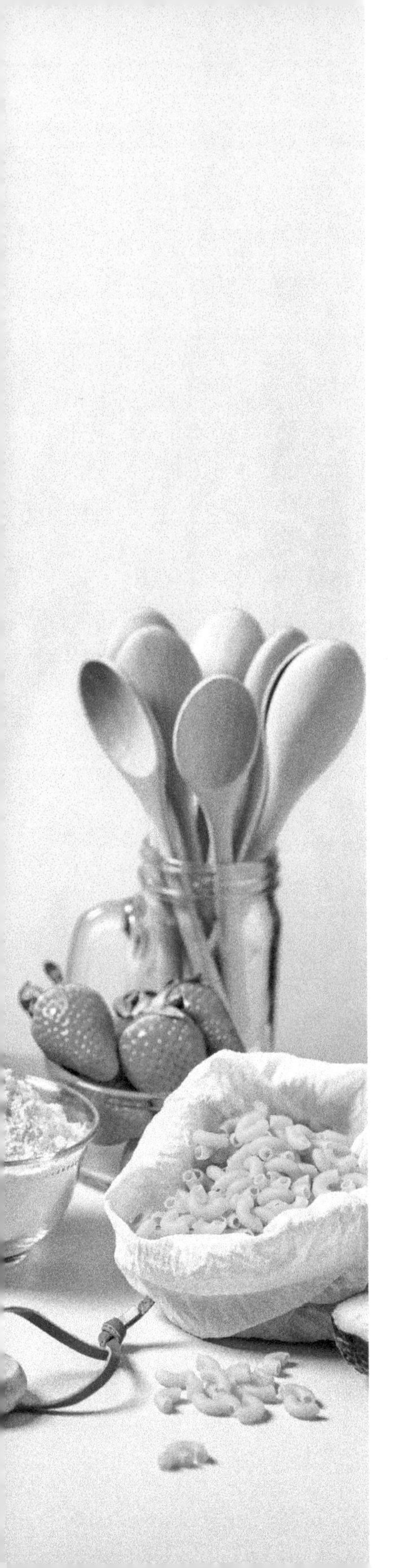

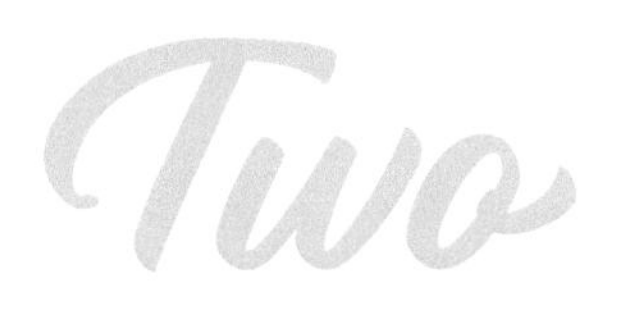

# Creating a Dairy-Free Kitchen

It's time to prep your kitchen for your new dairy-free lifestyle. Okay, so you won't be filling up your cheese drawer or butter compartment with your old standbys, but there's a whole world of delicious dairy-free foods at your disposal. From the countless foods that are naturally dairy-free, like fruits, vegetables, and meats, to dairy-free substitutes, you'll be able to stock your kitchen with everything needed for culinary success.

As you start to explore some of the dairy-free substitutes, don't expect them to taste exactly the same as their dairy counterparts. Instead, appreciate the substitutes for their own flavors, textures, and uses. You may find that you like some of them more than the dairy-filled versions!

You'll also find that some substitutes and recipes require new cooking techniques or adjustments, but these will be simple and doable even with limited cooking experience.

## Kitchen Cleanse

If everyone in your household is embarking on the dairy-free journey, it makes sense to purge all the dairy-filled items from your kitchen. Do a quick inventory of your fridge, freezer, and pantry. Get rid of both the obvious dairy products as well as any of the sneaky sources mentioned in chapter 1 (see page 5). This will help prevent any unintentional slipups—after all, it's easy to forget that a certain snack food or dressing has dairy in it, especially when you're in a hurry!

That said, sometimes only one individual—like you or your child—needs to follow a dairy-free diet. In this case, you may want to leave the dairy foods for the rest of the family. If you have a young child who does not quite understand the complexity of an allergy, make sure these dairy foods are out of reach to avoid accidental exposure.

## Stocking Your Pantry

Stocking your dairy-free kitchen doesn't need to be complicated. Start by loading up your grocery cart with all your favorite fruits, vegetables, meat, seafood, whole grains, beans, nuts, seeds, and oils. All of these foods, as long as they are minimally processed, are typically dairy-free.

You'll also want to keep these dairy-free kitchen staples on hand:

- **Cashews:** Soaked cashews processed in a food processor provide a creamy base for many dishes, including Scallion Cream Cheese (page 35).
- **Canned coconut milk:** From homemade whipped cream to savory curries, coconut milk is versatile for cooking both sweet and savory dishes.
- **Mayonnaise:** Mayo provides a creaminess and rich mouthfeel in several recipes, like homemade Ranch Dressing (page 39) and Mexican Street Corn (page 82).

- **Nutritional yeast:** This ingredient adds a lovely savory, cheesy flavor to dishes like pasta or popcorn. Some major grocery stores stock it in the natural foods section, but if you can't find it there, try a natural foods store or online retailer.
- **Vegan butter:** Vegan butter has a rich, buttery taste and is a must-have for many dairy-free desserts.
- **Vinegar:** Different types of vinegar are helpful to keep on hand for recipes such as homemade "buttermilk," dressings, and marinades.

## GREAT SNACKSPECTATIONS

Craving a midday dairy-free munchie? Keep these easy, energy-packed snacks on hand:

Sliced vegetables and guacamole

Pita bread and hummus

Hard-boiled eggs

Ants on a log (celery, peanut butter, and raisins)

Fresh fruit

Homemade trail mix (nuts, seeds, and dried fruit)

Frozen grapes

Roasted chickpeas

Rice cakes with nut butter

Tuna and dairy-free crackers

Beef jerky

## Equipment Must-Haves

In addition to stocking your kitchen with the right foods, it's also helpful to have a few key pieces of equipment on hand:

- **Baking sheets:** From sheet pan dinners to cookies, baking sheets are a must-have for any kitchen.
- **Blender:** When preparing smoothies or plant-based milks, a blender is vital.
- **Fine-mesh sieve:** If you plan to make your own milks, you'll need a fine-mesh sieve or cheesecloth to strain the pulp from the nuts, oats, or seeds.
- **Silicone baking mats:** These ensure your final product doesn't stick to the pan or over-brown on the bottom. You can also use parchment paper instead.
- **Stand or hand mixer:** It's not a necessity, but if you love baking, a mixer will help you quickly and easily blend batters and doughs for your favorite dairy-free treats.

## How to Cook Without Dairy

Cooking without dairy can be as simple as choosing recipes that are naturally dairy-free, or you can experiment with modifying recipes using simple swaps (like using dairy-free yogurt instead of regular yogurt). A third option is to create your own homemade dairy-free essentials to use in cooking, like the recipes found in chapter 3, or you can purchase them at the store instead.

Keep these helpful tips in mind as you flex your culinary muscles:

**Embrace both "new" and "tried and true."** Even if you're just starting this diet, it's possible that you are already comfortable cooking at least a few naturally dairy-free meals. For example, is there a stir-fry recipe your family loves? Do you enjoy meat and veggie kebabs on the grill? What about a big bowl of jambalaya? Make a list of all the meals you enjoy that are already free of dairy ingredients. When you create a meal plan for the week, include a few items from this "tried and true" list, along with a couple of new recipes. This will make your week less overwhelming than cooking new dishes every single night.

**Use simple swaps.** Most recipes and snacks can be made dairy-free with very easy swaps. If you love a bowl of cereal each morning, continue that tradition using a plant-based milk. Enjoy a midday sandwich? No problem. Skip the cheese and add smashed avocado or tapenade instead. Can't help digging into ice cream on Friday nights? Swap it out for a dairy-free version made from oats, cashews, or coconut—or try sorbet.

**Keep vegan butter on hand for baking.** Whether you're whipping up a batch of dairy-free cookies or cupcakes, vegan butter is a staple for all your baking needs. Find it at the store in both tubs and sticks, and substitute it in a 1:1 ratio for regular butter. With this trick, you can easily modify your favorite dessert recipes to fit your new dairy-free lifestyle.

**Choose the right plant-based milk for your dish.** With so many available options, it can be tough deciding which nondairy milk to choose for your recipes. Because each has a different taste, texture, and fat content, you'll want to choose the best fit for the type of dish you're making. Here are a few suggestions, depending on what you plan to make:

- **Sweet desserts:** almond milk, cashew milk, oat milk, rice milk, soy milk
- **Pancakes and waffles:** almond milk, oat milk, soy milk, hemp milk, flax milk
- **Soups, sauces, and savory dishes:** hemp milk, flax milk, cashew milk, soy milk, canned coconut milk
- **Homemade whipped cream:** canned coconut milk or coconut cream
- **Over cereal, drinking plain, or in smoothies:** almond milk, cashew milk, flax milk, oat milk, soy milk, coconut milk beverage (not canned)
- **In coffee:** dairy-free creamers, barista-style oat milk, soy milk

**Experiment with dairy-free cheeses.** Dairy-free cheeses vary considerably in taste, texture, and meltability. Because they lack the high fat content and rich flavor of traditional cheese, it may take a little experimenting to find the one or two you enjoy best.

Consider splurging on several different options and conducting your own at-home taste test. Experiment with cheeses made from different bases, like soy versus nuts, as well as different flavors across brands. You're sure to find at least a few options you enjoy!

Also try using the cheeses in different ways, from sampling as is, to melting on a pizza, to mixing in a casserole. Some cheeses may taste great melted in a dish, but aren't as appetizing cold on a cracker—or vice versa.

**Read every label.** When grocery shopping for your meals, read the ingredients on any packaged products to confirm they're dairy-free. Whole foods, such as fresh fruits, vegetables, and whole cuts of meat, are consistently safe choices, but processed foods require a quick sweep of the ingredients label each time you purchase them. Even if a food was previously safe, a manufacturer can change their formulations at any time.

Although this seems like extra work, the flip side is that you'll be pleasantly surprised at some of the foods that are dairy-free. For example, would you believe that some brands of refrigerated pie crusts, packaged frostings, and brownie mixes are naturally dairy-free? It's true! By becoming a label reader, you'll come to understand just how far you can stretch your culinary horizons.

## 7-Day Meal Plan

Meal planning involves writing down a list of recipes for the week, then grocery shopping and cooking based on that list. This will help you stick to your new diet, ease dinnertime stress, and save money on groceries. With just an hour or two of planning and shopping on the weekend, you'll know exactly what to make each night of the week and have all the ingredients you need on hand.

To make your own meal plan, jot down the dinners you plan to make each night. Then fill in breakfast, lunch, and snack ideas. For some people, it might be enough to just always have cereal, plant-based milk, and eggs on their list for breakfast. Others may want a different breakfast each day. Approach this in a way that works for you and your family.

Here's a sample meal plan:

### Day 1:

**Breakfast:** Meal Prep Egg Muffins with Butternut Squash and Sausage (page 52)

**Lunch:** Barbecue Beef Salad (page 67)

**Snack:** Classic Hummus (page 85) with vegetables for dipping

**Dinner:** Sheet Pan Salmon and Veggies (page 118)

**Breakfast:** Sunshine Smoothie (page 45)

**Lunch:** Leftover Barbecue Beef Salad

**Snack:** Frozen Banana Bites (page 90)

**Dinner:** Portobello Sheet Pan Fajitas (page 102)

## Day 3:

**Breakfast:** Leftover Meal Prep Egg Muffins

**Lunch:** Leftover Portobello Sheet Pan Fajitas

**Snack:** Leftover Frozen Banana Bites

**Dinner:** Korean Ground Beef Bowls (page 143)

## Day 4:

**Breakfast:** Raspberry-Chocolate Overnight Oats (page 46)

**Lunch:** Curried Tuna Salad Pita Pocket (page 114)

**Snack:** Classic Hummus (page 85) with vegetables for dipping

**Dinner:** Easy Turkey Meatloaf (page 137) and vegetables

### Day 5:

**Breakfast:** Sunshine Smoothie (page 45)

**Lunch:** Leftover Easy Turkey Meatloaf and vegetables

**Snack:** Chili-Lime Popcorn (page 88)

**Dinner:** Cauliflower and Sweet Potato Tacos (page 99)

### Day 6:

**Breakfast:** Raspberry-Chocolate Overnight Oats (page 46)

**Lunch:** Curried Tuna Salad Pita Pocket (page 114)

**Snack:** Leftover Chili-Lime Popcorn

**Dinner:** Lemony White Bean and Orzo Soup (page 72)

### Day 7:

**Breakfast:** Belgian Waffles (page 49)

**Lunch:** Leftover Lemony White Bean and Orzo Soup

**Snack:** Leftover Frozen Banana Bites

**Dinner:** Barbecue Chicken Pizza (page 132)

## Suggested Special Occasion Menus

When holidays or special occasions roll around, you may feel a little bummed out if you're not able to snag a bite of your grandmother's famous cream pie or make your favorite eggnog recipe. But don't you worry; this book has you covered with dairy-free foods that are perfect for any occasion! When you whip up these dishes, everyone—including you—can dig in, happily and worry-free.

### OCCASION: *BIRTHDAY PARTY*

Frosted Sugar Cookie Bars (page 150)

Chocolate Cake with Marshmallow Buttercream Frosting (page 160)

Pineapple-Coconut Ice Pops (page 153)

Chili-Lime Popcorn (page 88)

### OCCASION: *THANKSGIVING*

Pumpkin and Apple Soup (page 70)

Creamy Mashed Potatoes (page 83) with Mushroom and Sweet Onion Gravy (page 77)

Balsamic Honey Collard Greens (page 79)

Pumpkin Pie (page 157)

### OCCASION: *FOURTH OF JULY*

BLT Pasta Salad (page 62)

Southwestern Turkey Burgers (page 136)

Mexican Street Corn (page 82)

Strawberry Shortcake (page 155)

OCCASION: *BRUNCH WITH FRIENDS OR FAMILY*

Biscuits with Whipped Blueberry Butter Spread (page 47)

Bagels with Scallion Cream Cheese (page 35)

Potato, Bacon, and Apple Hash (page 51)

Fried Chicken (page 130) over Belgian Waffles (page 49)

OCCASION: *WINTER HOLIDAY PARTY*

French Onion Dip (page 86) with chips or veggies

Bacon-Wrapped Green Beans (page 80)

Hungarian Cookies (page 151)

Cinnamon Sugar Biscuit Donuts (page 158)

## About the Recipes

This cookbook is geared toward beginners, with easy-to-follow recipes. Many require minimal ingredients and/or short cooking times, and are manageable even if you have limited cooking experience. You'll find options that are nutritious and indulgent, and you'll never feel like you can't enjoy your favorite foods!

In addition, all the recipes include bonus tips, like how to substitute an uncommon ingredient or change up the flavor profile. Even if you have all the ingredients on hand and plan to make the recipe as written, give these tips a glance, as they can help inspire future meal ideas.

Every recipe in this cookbook is dairy-free. But some recipes also have labels for other restrictions that you may wish to follow. The following labels appear on recipes when applicable:

**Vegetarian/Vegan:** Recipes labeled vegetarian do not contain meat, poultry, or fish. Recipes labeled vegan do not contain any animal products, including meat, fish, eggs, and honey.

If a vegan recipe calls for ingredients that are also available in nonvegan variants, such as some brands of refined sugars, it's assumed you're purchasing a vegan-friendly option.

**Gluten-free:** These recipes do not contain wheat or overt gluten ingredients. Recipes with oats and oat milk will be labeled gluten-free, but be sure you are purchasing certified gluten-free varieties if you are on a gluten-free diet. Check labels on any processed ingredients (for example, vegan butter) to ensure that it's gluten-free.

**Soy-free:** Does not contain soy foods like tofu, edamame, soy sauce, etc. For recipes labeled soy-free that include vegan butter, dairy-free cheese, or dairy-free chocolate, it is assumed you are purchasing soy-free varieties. Check labels on any other processed ingredients as well.

**Nut-free:** Does not contain peanuts or tree nuts. For recipes labeled nut-free that include processed ingredients (e.g., vegan butter or dairy-free cheese), it is assumed you are purchasing nut-free varieties. A nut-free recipe can, however, contain coconut. Although the FDA lumps coconut into the tree nut category for allergen labeling, botanically coconut is a fruit. In addition, a coconut allergy is actually quite rare. If you have a tree nut allergy, talk to your doctor prior to consuming recipes with coconut.

**Egg-free:** Does not contain eggs or egg-based ingredients (for example, mayonnaise).

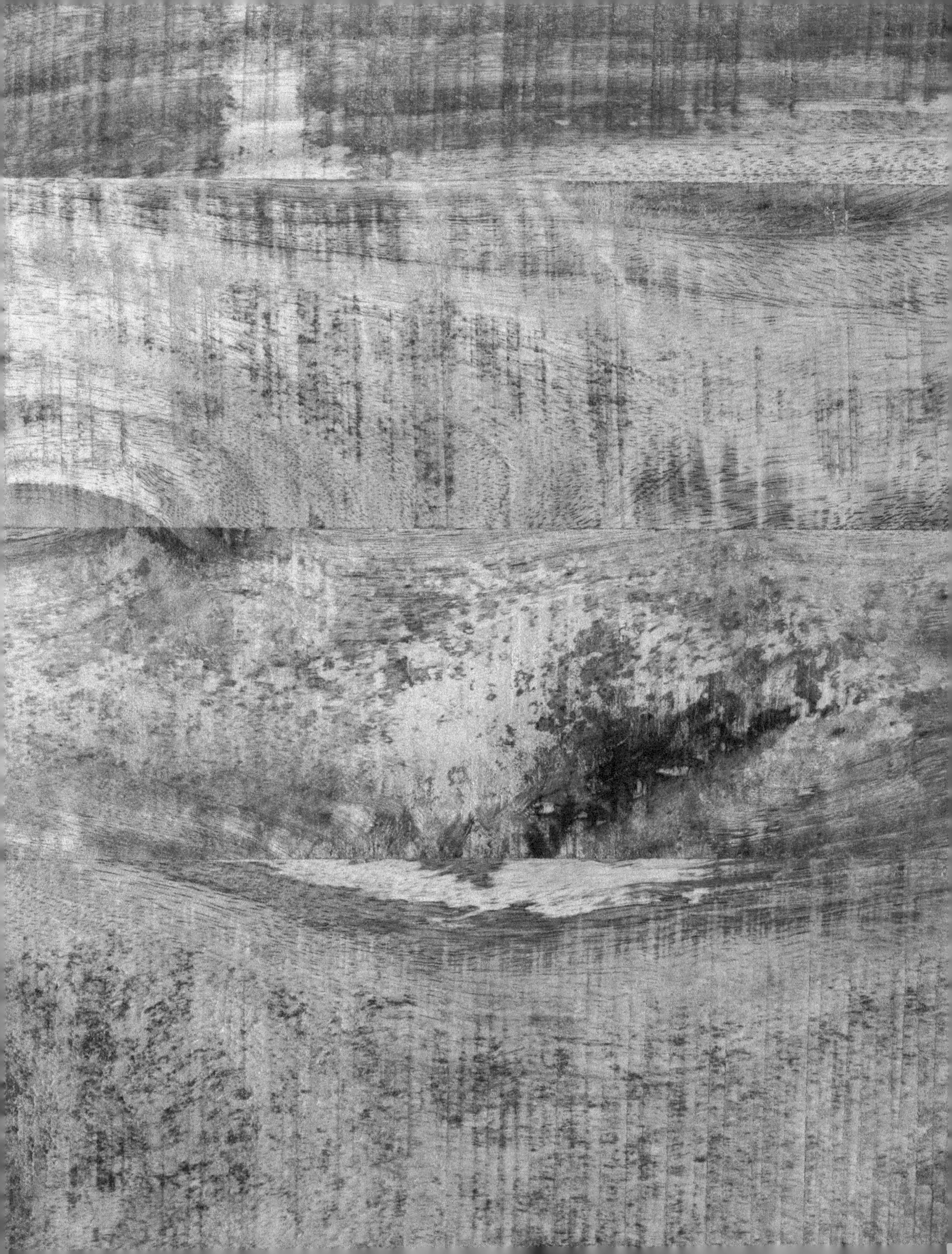

## Coconut Whipped Cream

*page 40*

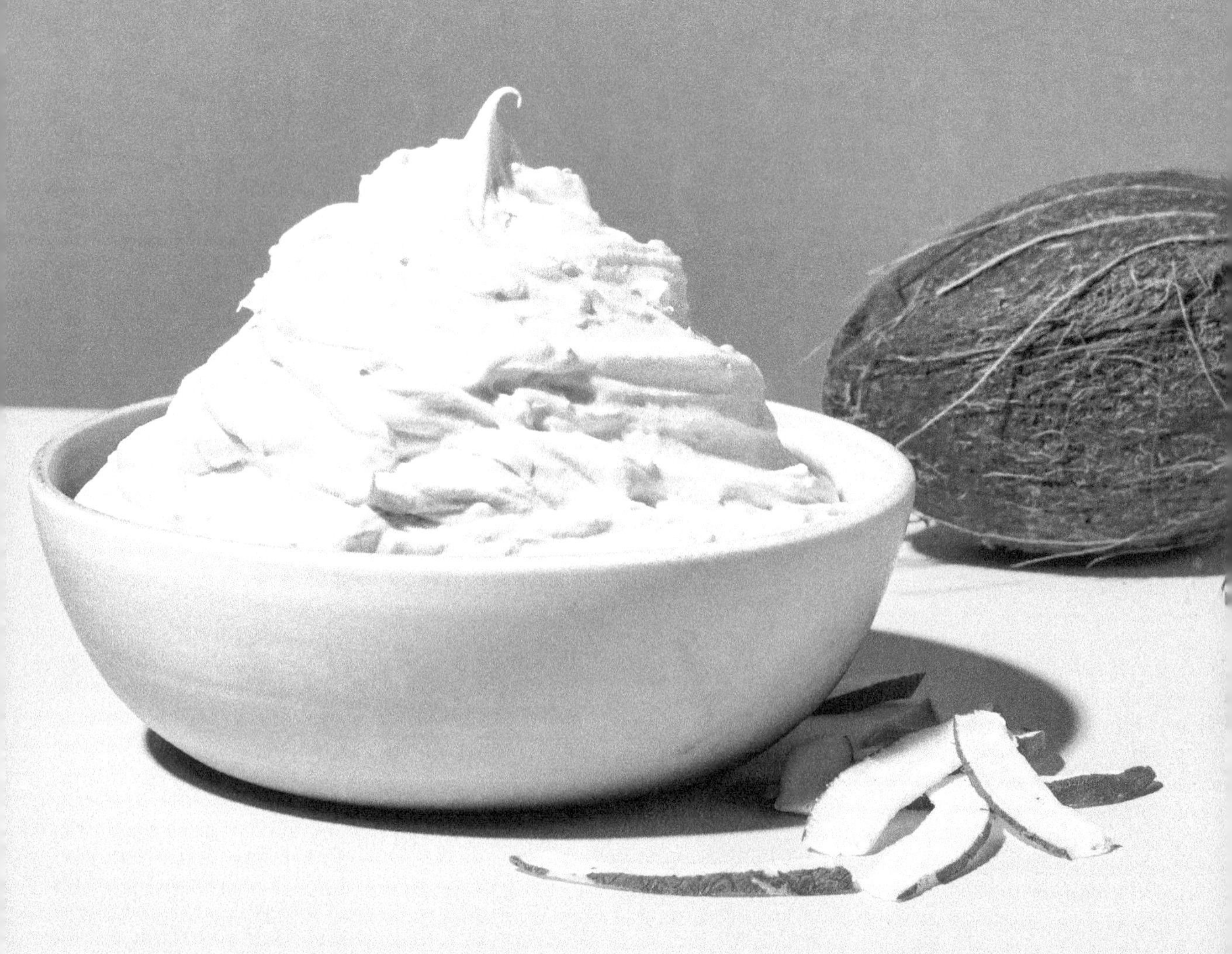

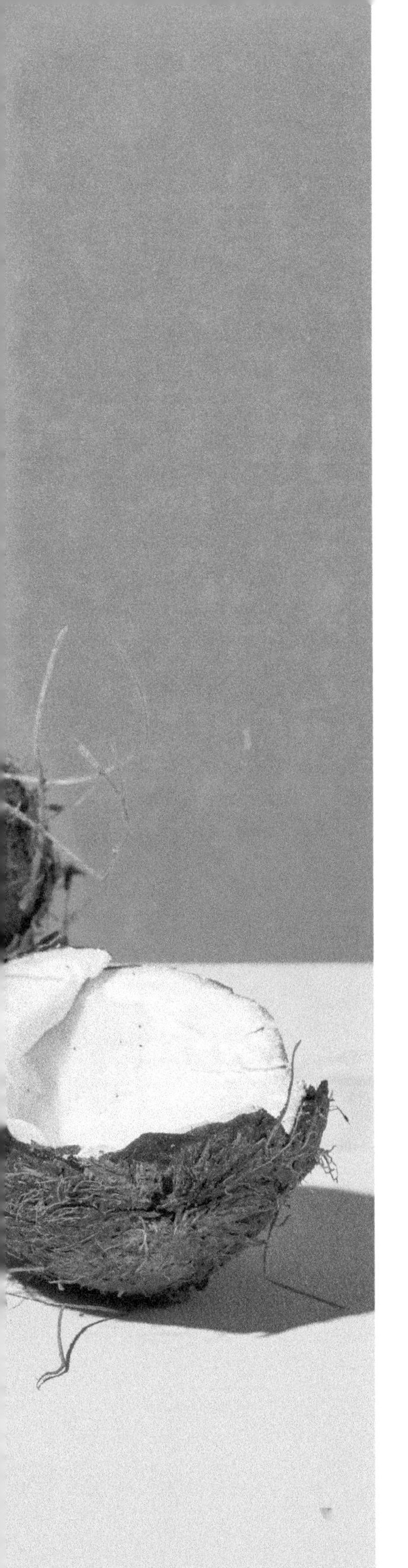

Three

# Dairy-Free Essentials (Milks, Cheeses, and Creams)

# ALMOND MILK

**Makes 1 quart**
**Prep time: 10 minutes, plus overnight to soak**

*Egg-Free, Gluten-Free, Soy-Free, Vegetarian*

As one of the most versatile plant-based milks, almond milk is one you'll always want to have on hand. You can easily grab a carton from the store, but if you'd prefer a less processed version, try this recipe. If you have a high-powered blender, you can pulverize and extract more of the almonds into the milk, resulting in a better taste. Leave this recipe unsweetened for cooking, or add vanilla and honey to make it more pleasant for drinking or serving over cereal.

1 cup raw almonds
4 cups water, plus more for soaking
⅛ teaspoon salt
½ teaspoon vanilla extract (optional)
1 to 2 tablespoons honey (optional)

1. Put the almonds in a large mason jar and add enough water to cover the nuts by a few inches. Cover and allow to soak in the refrigerator for at least 8 and up to 24 hours. Drain and rinse the almonds.

2. In a blender, combine the soaked almonds, 4 cups of water, salt, vanilla (if using), and honey (if using). Blend on high for 60 to 90 seconds. Set a fine-mesh sieve over a bowl and pour in the mixture (discard the pulp).

3. Transfer the milk to a covered container and store in the refrigerator for up to 4 days, stirring well before serving. If the milk separates, stir to recombine.

*Ingredient tip:* For a thicker almond milk, use heat: Follow the recipe, then pour half the mixture into a small pot. Over medium-high heat, heat the almond milk until almost at a boil. Remove from the heat and mix with the other half of the almond milk, then refrigerate. It will thicken as it cools, creating a creamier milk.

*Protein swap:* Use this same basic recipe for other nut-based milks. Just swap out the almonds for cashews, macadamia nuts, Brazil nuts, or pistachios.

---

**Per Serving (1 cup):** Calories: 30; Total fat: 2.5g; Carbohydrates: 1g; Cholesterol: 0mg; Fiber: 1g; Protein: 1g; Sugar: 0g

# OAT MILK

**Makes 1 quart**
**Prep time: 10 minutes**

*Egg-Free, Nut-Free, Soy-Free, Vegan, Gluten-Free Option*

Homemade oat milk is delectably thick and creamy, and probably the most cost-efficient dairy-free milk you can find. You can make it with just oats, water, and salt—but I recommend adding vanilla and dates for flavor and sweetness if you plan to enjoy it by the glass. One of the biggest complaints with homemade oat milk is its tendency to get slimy, but this can easily be prevented. Don't soak the oats ahead of time. You also want to blend for only 30 to 60 seconds, and avoid heating it for warm drinks. The same starch that makes for a creamy cup of hot oatmeal is still present in the milk, and heating can cause it to thicken up.

1 cup rolled oats (certified gluten-free if needed)
4 cups water
⅛ teaspoon salt
½ teaspoon vanilla extract (optional)
3 or 4 pitted dates (optional)

1. In a blender, combine the oats, water, salt, and vanilla (if using) and/or dates (if using) and blend for 30 to 60 seconds. Strain the liquid through a fine-mesh sieve or cheesecloth into a pitcher (discard the oat pulp).
2. Cover and store refrigerated for up to 5 days, stirring well before serving. If the milk separates, stir to recombine.

*Substitution tip:* If you don't have pitted dates on hand, sweeten with a few tablespoons of maple syrup, agave nectar, or honey.

---

**Per Serving (1 cup):** Calories: 100; Total fat: 1.5g; Carbohydrates: 18g; Cholesterol: 0mg; Fiber: 2g; Protein: 4g; Sugar: 5g

# CHOCOLATE CASHEW MILK

**Makes 1 quart**
**Prep time: 15 minutes, plus overnight to soak**

With its slightly nutty flavor and creamy texture, cashew milk is a perfect choice for homemade chocolate milk. I recommend using cheesecloth, a nut milk bag, or even a clean, old T-shirt to strain this recipe, rather than a fine-mesh strainer. Cashew pieces break down smaller than other nuts and often pass through fine mesh, leading to grainy milk. The other straining tools create the ultimate silky chocolate beverage.

**For the cashew milk**
1 cup raw cashews
4 cups water, divided, plus more for soaking
⅛ teaspoon salt
¼ cup pure maple syrup
¼ teaspoon ground cinnamon
½ teaspoon vanilla extract

**For the chocolate sauce**
¼ cup unsweetened cocoa powder
4 to 5 tablespoons hot water

**To make the cashew milk:** Put the cashews in a mason jar and add enough water to cover the nuts by a few inches. Cover and soak in the refrigerator for at least 8 and up to 24 hours. Drain and rinse the cashews.

In a blender, combine the soaked cashews and 2 cups of water. Blend for about 30 seconds, until the mixture looks fairly smooth.

Add the remaining 2 cups of water, salt, maple syrup, cinnamon, and vanilla. Blend for another 30 seconds.

Strain the mixture through a cheesecloth into a pitcher (discard the pulp).

**To make the chocolate sauce:** Put the cocoa powder in a small bowl. Add the hot water, 1 tablespoon at a time, whisking until you have a liquid chocolate syrup.

Pour the syrup into the pitcher of cashew milk, whisking well. Store covered in the refrigerator for up to 4 days, stirring well before serving.

*Make it easier:* Although it's tempting to toss the cocoa powder directly into the cashew milk to save time, the powder will clump together. Stirring in the liquid syrup ensures a well-blended chocolate milk. You can also buy a dairy-free chocolate syrup at the store. Skip the maple syrup in the cashew-milk base, and use the store-bought chocolate syrup to flavor and sweeten your cashew milk.

---

**Per Serving (1 cup):** Calories: 112; Total fat: 4.5g; Carbohydrates: 19g; Cholesterol: 0mg; Fiber: 2g; Protein: 2g; Sugar: 12g

# DAIRY-FREE BUTTERMILK

**Makes 1 cup**
**Prep time: 5 minutes**

*Egg-Free, Gluten-Free, Vegan, Nut-Free Option, Soy-Free Option*

Whether you need buttermilk for a pancake recipe or Fried Chicken (page 130), it's easy to make your own dairy-free version. Decide which plant-based milk to use based on the dish you're preparing. For sweeter desserts, you'll want to use an unsweetened or sweetened almond, oat, or soy milk. For savory dishes, try unsweetened almond milk, flax milk, hemp milk, or soy milk. Don't use canned coconut milk, as the fat content will be too high for most recipes that call for buttermilk.

1 cup dairy-free milk
1 tablespoon distilled white vinegar

Pour the dairy-free milk into a liquid measuring cup. Add the vinegar and let the mixture sit for 5 minutes. Use this in any recipe that calls for buttermilk as a 1:1 substitution.

*Substitution tip:* If you don't have vinegar, you can also use 1 tablespoon of lemon juice.

---

**Per Serving (¼ cup):** Calories: 21; Total fat: 1.5g; Carbohydrates: 0.6g; Cholesterol: 0mg; Fiber: 0.6g; Protein: 0.6g; Sugar: 0g

# SCALLION CREAM CHEESE

**Serves 8**
**Prep time: 15 minutes, plus overnight to soak**

*Egg-Free, Gluten-Free, Soy-Free, Vegan*

Dairy-free cream cheese doesn't have the exact same taste and texture as its conventional counterpart, but you may find that you like this plant-based version even more! The scallions and onion powder give it a punch of flavor that tastes great spread on a bagel or toast, and the cashews create the smooth base for this cream cheese.

1 cup raw cashews
¼ cup coconut cream (from a 13.5-ounce can of coconut milk)
2 teaspoons distilled white vinegar
2 tablespoons fresh lemon juice
¼ teaspoon salt
1 teaspoon onion powder
2 or 3 scallions, chopped

1. Put the cashews in a mason jar and add enough water to cover the nuts by a few inches. Soak in the refrigerator for at least 8 and up to 24 hours. Drain and rinse the cashews. Place the can of coconut milk in the refrigerator for 8 to 24 hours as well, to allow the coconut cream to rise to the top and firm up.
2. Drain the cashews, then transfer them to a small food processor or high-powered blender. Open the coconut milk, spoon out ¼ cup of the cream from the top, and add to the food processor. Add the vinegar, lemon juice, salt, onion powder, and scallions.
3. Process in 30-second bursts, opening to stir as needed, for 1 to 3 minutes, until the mixture reaches a nice, smooth texture. Serve or store in the refrigerator for up to 4 days.

*Make it easier:* If you don't have time to do the overnight prep, soak the cashews by bringing them to a boil in a pot of water, then letting them sit for 30 minutes. Swap the coconut cream for 3 to 4 tablespoons of plain dairy-free yogurt.

---

**Per Serving (2 tablespoons):** Calories: 121; Total fat: 10g; Carbohydrates: 7g; Cholesterol: 0mg; Fiber: 1g; Protein: 4g; Sugar: 1g

# DAIRY-FREE PARMESAN

**Makes 10 tablespoons**
**Prep time: 5 minutes**

Parmesan cheese delivers a salty, savory element to many recipes–and you don't have to miss out on that with this dairy-free substitute. Ground cashews provide the textural base of the dish, and nutritional yeast and other seasonings add the cheesy, savory goodness. Use this as a delicious topping for pizza, pasta, or salads. Although many dairy-free essentials use raw cashews, I recommend using roasted cashews for this recipe.

- ½ cup unsalted roasted cashews
- 2 tablespoons nutritional yeast
- ¼ teaspoon garlic powder
- ¼ teaspoon salt
- ⅛ teaspoon onion powder

In a small food processor or high-powered blender, combine the cashews, nutritional yeast, garlic powder, salt, and onion powder and pulse several times until the texture looks similar to grated Parmesan cheese. Transfer to an airtight container and store in the refrigerator for up to 2 weeks.

*Substitution tip:* If you're allergic to nuts, you can make this recipe using ½ cup roasted hemp hearts in place of the cashews.

---

**Per Serving (1 tablespoon):** Calories: 43; Total fat: 3g; Carbohydrates: 3g; Cholesterol: 0mg; Fiber: 0.5g; Protein: 1g; Sugar: 0.5g

# ITALIAN-STYLE CASHEW RICOTTA

**Makes 1½ cups**
**Prep time: 10 minutes, plus 25 minutes to soak / Cook time: 5 minutes**

*Egg-Free, Gluten-Free, Soy-Free, Vegan*

From stuffed shells to lasagna, you'll want this cashew ricotta stand-in for all of your favorite Italian dishes. When processed with lemon juice, the cashews take on a thick, creamy texture reminiscent of traditional ricotta. Seasoning it with basil, oregano, and garlic amps up the flavor, and may even trick some into thinking it's the real thing!

1¾ cups raw cashews
Juice of 1 large lemon
½ teaspoon salt
2 teaspoons dried basil
2 teaspoons dried oregano
1 teaspoon dried minced garlic
2 to 4 tablespoons water, as needed

1. Put the cashews in a pot and fill with water. Bring to a boil and cook for 5 minutes, then remove from the heat and let soak for 25 minutes. Drain and rinse the cashews.
2. In a small food processor or high-powered blender, combine the cashews, lemon juice, salt, basil, oregano, and garlic and process until smooth, 1 to 3 minutes, stirring as needed. Adjust the thickness to your preference by adding a tablespoon of water at a time.
3. Store the mixture in an airtight container in the refrigerator for up to 4 days. If it thickens too much, stir in a splash of water to thin it out.

*Make it easier:* You can also soak the cashews overnight if you'd prefer, rather than using the boiling method.

---

**Per Serving (¼ cup):** Calories: 218; Total fat: 17g; Carbohydrates: 13g; Cholesterol: 0mg; Fiber: 6g; Protein: 6g; Sugar: 0g

# CASHEW SOUR CREAM

**Makes about 1⅓ cups**
**Prep time: 15 minutes, plus overnight to soak**

*Egg-Free, Gluten-Free, Soy-Free, Vegan*

It's hard to imagine a plate of nachos or a loaded baked potato without a big ol' dollop of sour cream. This dairy-free variety offers the same tanginess as the traditional version, but it's made from cashews instead of milk. This recipe works best when you're looking to add a tangy, cooling component to a dish, like on top of Vegan Bean Chili (page 111). For sweet baked goods that call for sour cream, using coconut cream as a substitute often works better. For a sour cream–style dip for veggies or chips, try the French Onion Dip (page 86) instead.

1 cup raw cashews
2 tablespoons fresh lemon juice
2 teaspoons apple cider vinegar
¼ teaspoon salt
⅓ to ½ cup water

1. Put the cashews in a mason jar and add enough water to cover the nuts by a few inches. Soak in the refrigerator for at least 8 and up to 24 hours. Drain and rinse the cashews.
2. In a small food processor or high-powered blender, combine the cashews, lemon juice, vinegar, and salt and process until relatively smooth, 1 to 3 minutes, stirring as needed.
3. Add ⅓ cup of water and process again for 30 seconds. Add a little more water if desired for a thinner sour cream, or leave as is for a thicker version. Store covered in the refrigerator for up to 4 days.

*Substitution tip:* You can use distilled white vinegar instead of cider vinegar.

---

**Per Serving (2 tablespoons):** Calories: 70; Total fat: 5g; Carbohydrates: 4g; Cholesterol: 0mg; Fiber: 0g; Protein: 2g; Sugar: 1g

# RANCH DRESSING

**Makes 1½ cups**
**Prep time: 10 minutes**

*Gluten-Free, Nut-Free, Vegetarian*

Ranch dressing has a funny history. Did you know it was invented by a plumber-turned-ranch-owner? Steve Henson purchased a dude ranch with his wife. While living at the aptly named Hidden Valley Ranch, he continued to perfect a buttermilk-style dressing, which he served to guests. The location became known for the iconic dressing. Although this dairy-free version isn't the same as the original, I like to think it pays homage to the classic flavors in Henson's version.

- 1 cup mayonnaise
- ½ cup unsweetened oat milk or other dairy-free milk
- 1 teaspoon apple cider vinegar
- 1½ tablespoons chopped fresh parsley
- 1½ tablespoons minced fresh chives
- ½ teaspoon Italian seasoning
- ¼ teaspoon garlic powder
- ¼ teaspoon onion powder
- ¼ teaspoon freshly ground black pepper
- ¼ teaspoon salt

In a screw-top jar, combine all the ingredients, seal, and shake until well blended. Enjoy immediately, or store in the refrigerator for up to 5 days.

*Mix it up:* Try using different fresh herbs according to your taste preferences. Substitute dill for the parsley for a nice change of pace. Or switch it up for cilantro when using the dressing on a Southwestern salad.

---

**Per Serving (2 tablespoons):** Calories: 24; Total fat: 14g; Carbohydrates: 0.2g; Cholesterol: 7mg; Fiber: 0.1g; Protein: 0.1g; Sugar: 0g

# COCONUT WHIPPED CREAM

**Makes 1 to 1½ cups**
**Prep time: 10 minutes, plus overnight to separate**

*Egg-Free, Gluten-Free, Nut-Free, Soy-Free, Vegan*

Coconut whipped cream adds an extra layer of flavor to pies and cakes, and makes an excellent option for dipping fresh fruit. With this recipe, a few key steps will ensure success: First, chill the mixer bowl to ensure the coconut cream whips up as it's meant to. Second, use canned full-fat coconut milk, not the kind in the carton, which is called coconut milk beverage. Also, skip over any lite coconut milks—they won't have enough fat to support the whipping process.

Coconut cream from 1 (13.5-ounce) can full-fat coconut milk
½ teaspoon vanilla extract
1 to 6 tablespoons powdered sugar or other sweetener of your choice

Place the can of coconut milk in the refrigerator for 8 to 24 hours.

Chill a large bowl and whisk attachment in the refrigerator for 30 minutes.

Scoop out the solidified coconut cream from the top half of the can of coconut milk and put the cream in the chilled bowl. Using a stand mixer or hand mixer, whisk for 1 to 3 minutes, until peaks form.

Whisk in the vanilla and powdered sugar, 1 tablespoon at a time, adjusting to your preferences. Eat immediately, or store covered in the refrigerator for 1 to 2 days.

*Make it easier:* I've found that the ease of the cream separating in the can overnight and the quality of the whipped cream are both highly dependent on the brand of coconut milk. If you don't get the right texture or taste the first time around, try experimenting with different brands. (I like 365 Everyday Value Organic Coconut Milk.)

*Ingredient tip:* Don't throw away the thinner coconut liquid left in the can. Save this in a jar in the refrigerator and use it to add a tropical flavor to smoothies.

---

**Per Serving (2 tablespoons/medium sweet):** Calories: 92; Total fat: 3.5g; Carbohydrates: 15g; Cholesterol: 0mg; Fiber: 0g; Protein: 0g; Sugar: 14g

# LEMON AQUAFABA WHIPPED CREAM

**Makes 2 to 3 cups**
**Prep time: 10 minutes**

*Egg-Free, Gluten-Free, Nut-Free, Soy-Free, Vegan*

If you avoid both dairy and coconut, you'll want to bookmark this whipped cream recipe. Aquafaba refers to the liquid from a can of beans, and although it sounds a bit kooky to make whipped cream with it, you'll find the texture to be very light and fluffy. Depending on the brand, it can have a slightly "beany" taste, but the lemon extract and powdered sugar help mask this. The cream of tartar helps the whipped cream hold its shape, and the oil gives it a richer mouthfeel. This whipped cream's lemon-forward taste makes it great for serving over fruit, pound cake, or scones.

- Liquid (aquafaba) from 1 (15-ounce) can no-salt-added chickpeas
- ¼ teaspoon plus ⅛ teaspoon cream of tartar
- 2 teaspoons lemon extract
- ½ cup powdered sugar, plus more if needed
- 1 tablespoon canola oil or other neutral-tasting oil

1. Pour the liquid from the can of chickpeas into a medium bowl. Using a hand mixer or stand mixer, whisk for 2 to 3 minutes on high speed, until light and fluffy.

2. Add all of the cream of tartar and the lemon extract and continue beating for 1 minute. Add the powdered sugar and oil and beat for another 3 to 5 minutes, until very fluffy. Taste and adjust with more sugar if needed. Serve immediately, or store covered in the refrigerator for up to a few hours. (It will not hold its form for longer than that.)

*Substitution tip:* You can also use the liquid from a can of small white beans or cannellini beans, rather than chickpeas.

---

**Per Serving (¼ cup):** Calories: 43; Total fat: 1.5g; Carbohydrates: 6g; Cholesterol: 0mg; Fiber: 0g; Protein: 0g; Sugar: 6g

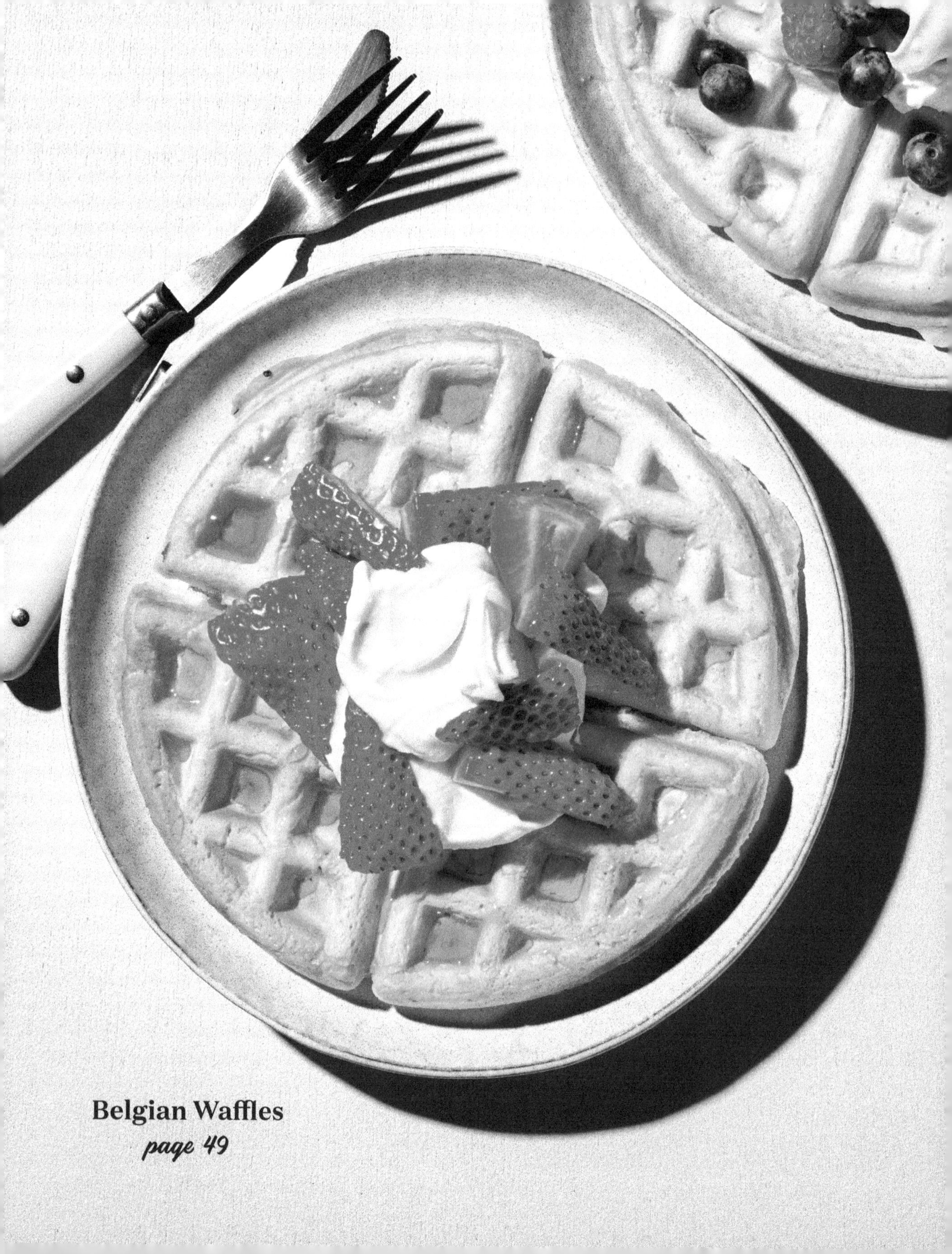

**Belgian Waffles**
*page 49*

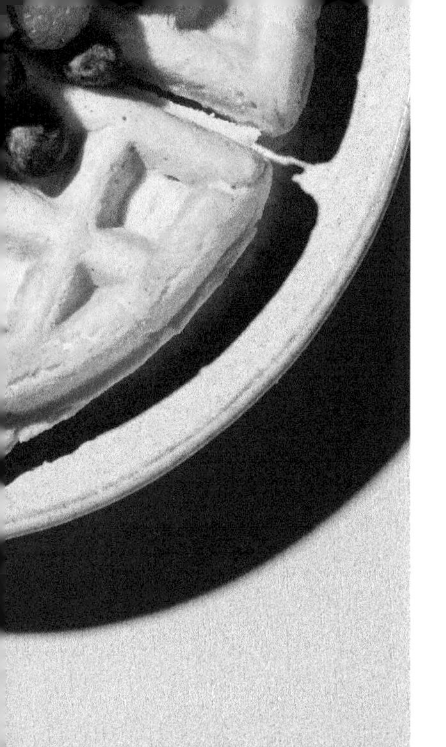

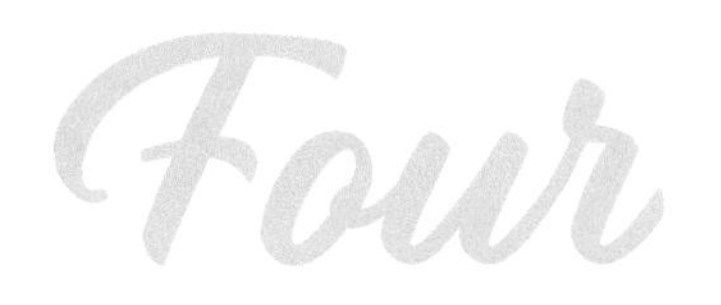


# Breakfast and Smoothies

# PINEAPPLE BANANA GREEN SMOOTHIE

**Makes 1 smoothie**
**Prep time: 5 minutes**

*Egg-Free, Gluten-Free, Nut-Free, Soy-Free, Vegan*

Adding more leafy greens to the day is a smart move for adults and kids alike. Spinach in particular contains beneficial compounds like vitamin K, which is involved in blood clotting, and lutein, a phytochemical linked to eye health. Smoothies are one of the easiest ways to boost your family's intake of leafy greens while simultaneously satisfying taste buds of all ages—especially since the pineapple and banana are all you taste!

- 1 cup canned juice-packed pineapple chunks
- ¼ cup pineapple juice (from the can)
- 1 medium banana, frozen in chunks
- ½ cup baby spinach
- ½ cup cold water

In a blender, combine the pineapple and pineapple juice. Add the frozen banana, spinach, and cold water and blend on high speed for about 30 seconds. Enjoy immediately.

*Mix it up:* Try using different greens, like kale or arugula. You can also change up the fruits, like substituting mango or strawberries for the pineapple.

---

**Per Serving (1 smoothie):** Calories: 294; Total fat: 0.5g; Carbohydrates: 75g; Cholesterol: 0mg; Fiber: 5.5g; Protein: 3g; Sugar: 57g

# SUNSHINE SMOOTHIE

**Makes 1 smoothie**
**Prep time: 5 minutes**

*Egg-Free, Nut-Free, Soy-Free, Vegan, Gluten-Free Option*

This smoothie will bring back memories of those orange cream ice pops from childhood. With bright orange and vanilla flavors, it's a delightful way to start your morning, but it can also double as a healthier dessert. If you choose to add the optional scoop of vanilla plant-based protein powder, it'll boost the protein content and make it more filling.

- 1 banana, frozen in chunks
- 1 clementine, peeled and halved
- ½ cup vanilla oat milk (certified gluten-free if needed)
- ½ cup orange juice
- 3 ice cubes
- 1 scoop vanilla plant-based protein powder (optional)

In a blender, combine all the ingredients and blend for about 30 seconds, until smooth. Enjoy immediately.

*Make it easier:* Some grocery stores offer markdowns on produce like overripe bananas. When you find these deals, grab a bunch, then chop and freeze them as soon as you get home. You'll always be prepared for smoothie time. (This is also a great use for the bananas that overripened on your counter!)

---

**Per Serving (1 smoothie):** Calories: 245; Total fat: 1.5g; Carbohydrates: 58g; Cholesterol: 0mg; Fiber: 5.5g; Protein: 4g; Sugar: 23g

# RASPBERRY-CHOCOLATE OVERNIGHT OATS

**Serves 1**

**Prep time: 10 minutes, plus overnight to soak**

*Egg-Free, Vegan, Gluten-Free Option, Nut-Free Option, Soy-Free Option*

Overnight oats are a convenient meal-prep breakfast that you can make on the weekend and enjoy for the next few mornings. The pairing of raspberries and dark chocolate used here is a classic sweet treat, yet this minimally sweetened oatmeal still meets my criteria for a healthy, nutritious breakfast.

- ½ cup rolled oats (certified gluten-free if needed)
- ½ cup unsweetened oat milk (certified gluten-free if needed) or other dairy-free milk
- ½ cup frozen raspberries
- ¼ cup plain dairy-free yogurt (soy-free or nut-free if needed)
- 2 tablespoons chia seeds
- 1 tablespoon dairy-free dark chocolate chips
- 1 teaspoon pure maple syrup

1. In a mason jar, combine all the ingredients and give everything a good shake to blend. Cover and refrigerate overnight.
2. In the morning, enjoy cold or warm. To heat, uncover and microwave for 60 to 90 seconds.

*Mix it up:* The base for any overnight oats recipe starts with just ½ cup rolled oats and ½ cup dairy-free milk. From there, mix it up any way you'd like. Try adding chopped kiwi, mango, and shredded coconut for a tropical version, or shredded carrots, nuts, and cinnamon for a carrot cake–style oatmeal.

---

**Per Serving:** Calories: 471; Total fat: 21g; Carbohydrates: 71g; Cholesterol: 0mg; Fiber: 21g; Protein: 14g; Sugar: 19g

# BISCUITS WITH WHIPPED BLUEBERRY BUTTER SPREAD

**Serves 8**

**Prep time: 15 minutes / Cook time: 15 minutes**

*Egg-Free, Soy-Free, Vegan*

A few years ago, I visited a bed-and-breakfast in Maine that served a delicious blueberry-infused butter with their dinner rolls. That was the inspiration for this dish. These dairy-free biscuits get their tender texture from cutting in cold vegan butter. The butter needs to stay solid in the dough before baking to achieve the best texture, so don't overwork the dough or let it sit very long. Work quickly to mix, cut them out, and get 'em in the oven.

**For the biscuits**

¾ cup unsweetened almond milk or other dairy-free milk
2 teaspoons distilled white vinegar
2 cups all-purpose flour, plus more for the work surface
1 tablespoon baking powder
1 tablespoon sugar
½ teaspoon salt
6 tablespoons cold vegan butter

**For the blueberry butter spread**

¼ cup frozen blueberries
8 tablespoons vegan butter
1 tablespoon pure maple syrup

1. **To make the biscuits:** Preheat the oven to 425°F. Line a baking sheet with a silicone baking mat or parchment paper.
2. In a glass, combine the almond milk and vinegar and set aside in the refrigerator for 5 minutes.
3. In a large bowl, combine the flour, baking powder, sugar, and salt. Cut in the cold butter until the mixture looks like coarse sand. Pour in the almond milk mixture and stir just until all ingredients are combined, being careful not to overmix. If the dough is too dry to hold together, add an extra tablespoon of almond milk at a time until it just comes together.
4. Transfer the dough to a lightly floured surface. Flatten into a disk about ¾ inch thick. Use a 3-inch biscuit cutter to cut 8 biscuits from the dough (gathering up the scraps if needed to get all 8) and place on the prepared baking sheet.
5. Bake for 14 to 16 minutes, or until light golden brown. Let cool slightly on the pan.

**To make the blueberry butter spread:** In a microwave-safe bowl, thaw the blueberries for 20 seconds. Add the butter and maple syrup to the bowl and beat with a hand mixer or stand mixer until light and fluffy.

Serve the warm biscuits with the blueberry butter spread.

*Make it easier:* Don't have time to make homemade biscuits? Check the refrigerated cans of biscuits in the dairy section at the grocery store–some are dairy-free!

---

**Per Serving:** Calories: 306; Total fat: 20g; Carbohydrates: 28g; Cholesterol: 0mg; Fiber: 1g; Protein: 3g; Sugar: 3.5g

# BELGIAN WAFFLES

**Makes 4 large waffles**
**Prep time: 15 minutes / Cook time: 15 minutes**

*Soy-Free, Vegetarian*

This yummy waffle recipe features pantry staples that you probably already have on hand. To retain crispiness after cooking the waffles, keep them in an oven set to 200°F until they're all cooked. Top them off with vegan butter and pure maple syrup, or fresh strawberries and Coconut Whipped Cream (page 40).

1½ cups unsweetened almond milk
1½ tablespoons fresh lemon juice
2 large eggs
3 tablespoons canola oil (or any oil of your choice)
2 tablespoons sugar
1 teaspoon vanilla extract
1¾ cups all-purpose flour
2 teaspoons baking powder
½ teaspoon salt

1. In a liquid measuring cup, combine the almond milk and lemon juice and let sit for 5 minutes.
2. In a large bowl, whisk together the eggs, oil, sugar, and vanilla. Add the almond milk mixture and whisk to make sure everything is well combined. Stir in the flour, baking powder, and salt.
3. Heat a Belgian waffle iron. When hot, pour in about ¾ cup of batter, then close the iron. Cook according to the manufacturer's directions (most have a light that turns on when done), usually 3 to 5 minutes each, or until the waffles are golden brown and crisp.

*Make it easier:* Save time by prepping a double batch of these on the weekend and then freezing the cooled leftovers in freezer-safe bags. Reheat one (or more) in an oven or toaster oven at 350°F for about 10 minutes, or until warm and crisp.

---

**Per Serving (1 waffle):** Calories: 363; Total fat: 14g; Carbohydrates: 49g; Cholesterol: 93mg; Fiber: 2g; Protein: 9g; Sugar: 6.5g

# MORNING GLORY BREAD

**Serves 10**
**Prep time: 15 minutes / Cook time: 40 minutes**

*Gluten-Free, Soy-Free, Vegetarian*

For a wholesome, nutritious breakfast, this morning glory bread is one of my top picks. It's naturally gluten-free, made with nutrient-dense almond flour, and is only lightly sweetened with a touch of honey. It's got wonderful flavor, though. Peanut butter gives this a subtle nuttiness, and it's packed with apple, carrots, coconut, and raisins, which offer a pleasant mixture of tastes and textures in each bite. Top a slice with vegan butter, jam, or your favorite nut butter.

- ½ cup peanut butter
- ¼ cup coconut oil, at room temperature, plus more for the pan
- ¼ cup honey
- 3 large eggs
- 1 teaspoon vanilla extract
- 2¼ cups almond flour
- 1½ teaspoons ground cinnamon
- 1 teaspoon baking soda
- ½ teaspoon salt
- 1 small apple, peeled, cored, and diced
- ¾ cup grated carrots
- ¼ cup unsweetened shredded coconut
- ¼ cup golden raisins

Preheat the oven to 350°F. Grease a 9-by-5-inch loaf pan with coconut oil.

In a large bowl, whisk together the peanut butter, coconut oil, honey, eggs, and vanilla until well combined. Stir in the almond flour, cinnamon, baking soda, and salt. Fold in the apple, carrots, coconut, and raisins.

Pour the batter into the prepared loaf pan. Bake for 40 to 45 minutes, or until the top is golden brown and a toothpick inserted in the center comes out clean. Enjoy immediately, or store in the refrigerator for up to 4 days.

*Mix it up:* Get creative with the add-ins for this bread. You can also try swapping in shredded zucchini, chopped pineapple, walnuts, or pecans.

---

**Per Serving:** Calories: 291; Total fat: 25g; Carbohydrates: 13g; Cholesterol: 0mg; Fiber: 4g; Protein: 8g; Sugar: 6.5g

# POTATO, BACON, AND APPLE HASH

**Serves 4 to 6**
**Prep time: 15 minutes / Cook time: 25 minutes**

*Egg-Free, Gluten-Free, Nut-Free, Soy-Free*

This breakfast hash combines savory russet potatoes and bacon with the sweeter elements of apples and sweet potatoes. The pairing is tasty, filling, and free of the eight allergens (see page 4). Make it ahead of time on the weekend for an easy grab-and-go dish later in the week.

2 medium sweet potatoes
2 medium russet potatoes
5 thick-cut bacon slices
2 small apples, peeled, cored, and chopped
¼ teaspoon salt
¼ teaspoon freshly ground black pepper
Olive oil, as needed

1. Rinse and scrub the sweet potatoes and russet potatoes. Poke each a few times with a fork, then place them in a microwave-safe bowl. Cook them in the microwave for 7 to 9 minutes, or until they start to get tender. When cool enough to handle, cut into bite-size pieces.
2. Meanwhile, in a large skillet, cook the bacon over medium heat until crisp. Transfer the bacon to paper towels to drain, leaving the bacon grease in the skillet.
3. Add the chopped potatoes, apples, salt, and pepper to the skillet. Cook over medium heat for about 10 minutes, adding olive oil as needed to help crisp up the potatoes and prevent them from sticking. When the potatoes have crisped up a bit on the outside and the apples are tender, remove from the heat.
4. Crumble the bacon and add it to the skillet. Give everything a good toss and enjoy warm.

*Mix it up:* Swap out the russet potatoes for fried yellow plantains for a sweeter, unconventional version of this hash. Peel and slice the plantain into ¼-inch-thick rounds and add them to the pan when you add the sweet potatoes and apples.

---

**Per Serving:** Calories: 292; Total fat: 13g; Carbohydrates: 39g; Cholesterol: 16mg; Fiber: 4.5g; Protein: 8g; Sugar: 11g

# MEAL PREP EGG MUFFINS WITH BUTTERNUT SQUASH AND SAUSAGE

**Makes 12 egg muffins**
**Prep time: 15 minutes / Cook time: 35 minutes**

*Gluten-Free, Nut-Free, Soy-Free*

When you have a busy week ahead, make a batch of these meal prep egg muffins on the weekend. You can store them in the fridge and pull out a couple each morning. Just microwave them to reheat, and breakfast is ready! Alternatively, these are excellent to whip up for a brunch with family or friends, along with a side of Biscuits with Whipped Blueberry Butter Spread (page 47).

1½ tablespoons olive oil, plus more for the pan
1 small yellow onion, chopped
1 bell pepper (any color), chopped
1¾ cups peeled butternut squash cubes (1/2 inch)
6 ounces breakfast sausage links (check to ensure dairy-free)
2 cups packed baby spinach
9 large eggs

1. Preheat the oven to 350°F. Thoroughly grease 12 cups of a muffin tin with olive oil.

2. Meanwhile, in a large skillet, heat the 1½ tablespoons of olive oil over medium heat. Add the onion, bell pepper, squash, and sausage links. Cover and cook for 5 minutes, then uncover and cook for an additional 10 minutes, until the squash is tender and the sausage links are cooked through. Stir in the spinach and cook for another minute, until it is lightly wilted. Remove the pan from the heat.

3. Remove the sausage links from the pan and chop into bite-size pieces. Toss back into the pan with the vegetables.

4. Crack the eggs into a large bowl and whisk until blended. Add the vegetables and sausage to the egg mixture. Divide the mixture evenly among the prepared muffin cups, filling them almost all the way to the top. Bake for 20 to 25 minutes, or until a knife comes out clean.

5. Enjoy warm. Store leftovers in the refrigerator for up to 4 days. To reheat, place two egg muffins in the microwave and cook for 30 to 60 seconds, until hot.

*Mix it up:* Customize these egg muffins to include whatever vegetable and meat combinations you prefer. Just swap out the veggies and sausage for ingredients you'd like to try. For a spicy kick, try jalapeños and browned ground beef, topped with salsa. Or try a vegetarian batch with sautéed kale and roasted red peppers.

---

**Per Serving (2 egg muffins):** Calories: 261; Total fat: 18g; Carbohydrates: 8g; Cholesterol: 303mg; Fiber: 2g; Protein: 16g; Sugar: 2.5g

# LOADED BAGEL BREAKFAST SANDWICH

**Makes 1 sandwich**
**Prep time: 5 minutes / Cook time: 5 minutes**

My son knows one of the first spots we check in the grocery store is the day-old bread shelf. Whenever we spot bakery-style bagels there that still feel soft, we grab them to stock up and freeze. Once they're frozen, you can pull them out for weeks to come to make tasty breakfast sandwiches whenever the craving strikes. Just pop one in the microwave for 30 to 45 seconds, then toast it, and it's ready to load up with your favorite ingredients. This particular combination of eggs, apples, arugula, and dairy-free cream cheese creates a lovely balance of sweet and savory elements.

- 1 large egg
- 1 bagel (check to ensure dairy-free)
- 2 tablespoons Scallion Cream Cheese (page 35)
- ⅓ apple, peeled, cored, and sliced
- ⅓ cup baby arugula

1. Place a small skillet over medium heat. Coat it with cooking spray, then fry the egg to your desired doneness.
2. Toast the bagel, then spread on the scallion cream cheese. Top with the sliced apple, arugula, and fried egg.

*Mix it up:* Try one of these other two tasty bagel sandwich combinations: peach butter or apple butter, eggs, arugula, and caramelized onions; or Scallion Cream Cheese, cucumbers, mashed avocado, and spinach.

---

**Per Serving (1 sandwich):** Calories: 518; Total fat: 15g; Carbohydrates: 75g; Cholesterol: 186mg; Fiber: 4.5g; Protein: 21g; Sugar: 21g

# STEAK AND BEAN BREAKFAST BURRITOS

**Makes 5 burritos**
**Prep time: 15 minutes / Cook time: 20 minutes**

*Egg-Free, Nut-Free*

Most people get plenty of protein at dinner, but here you'll switch things up with a protein-packed breakfast burrito. The combination of steak, beans, veggies, and salsa creates a filling morning meal that won't leave you hungry an hour later. This recipe uses my favorite cast iron skillet cooking method to achieve a perfect medium-rare steak, but you can also grill the steak instead.

2 tablespoons olive oil, divided
1 pound petite sirloin steak
¼ teaspoon salt
1 medium yellow onion, sliced
1 bell pepper (any color), sliced
5 burrito-size flour tortillas
½ cup canned black beans, rinsed and drained
1 avocado, chopped
5 tablespoons salsa

1. In a cast iron skillet, heat 1 tablespoon of oil over medium heat. Season the steak with the salt, then add to the pan and let cook for 5 minutes on one side. Flip and cook for an additional 3 to 5 minutes, depending on thickness. Transfer the steak to a plate and cover loosely with aluminum foil. Let rest for 10 minutes.

2. Meanwhile, heat the remaining 1 tablespoon of oil in the same skillet. Sauté the onion and bell pepper for 6 to 8 minutes, or until tender. Remove from the heat.

3. Slice the steak into bite-size pieces and divide evenly among the tortillas. Add some onions, peppers, beans, avocado, and salsa to each tortilla. Wrap up and enjoy.

*Make it easier:* You can prep the ingredients for this ahead of time. However, don't put the burritos together until you plan to eat them, or they'll get soggy.

*Protein swap:* Not in the mood for steak? Swap in scrambled eggs instead for a vegetarian version of this recipe.

---

**Per Serving (1 burrito):** Calories: 455; Total fat: 18g; Carbohydrates: 45g; Cholesterol: 63mg; Fiber: 5g; Protein: 29g; Sugar: 3.5g

Crunchy Broccoli Salad

*page 60*

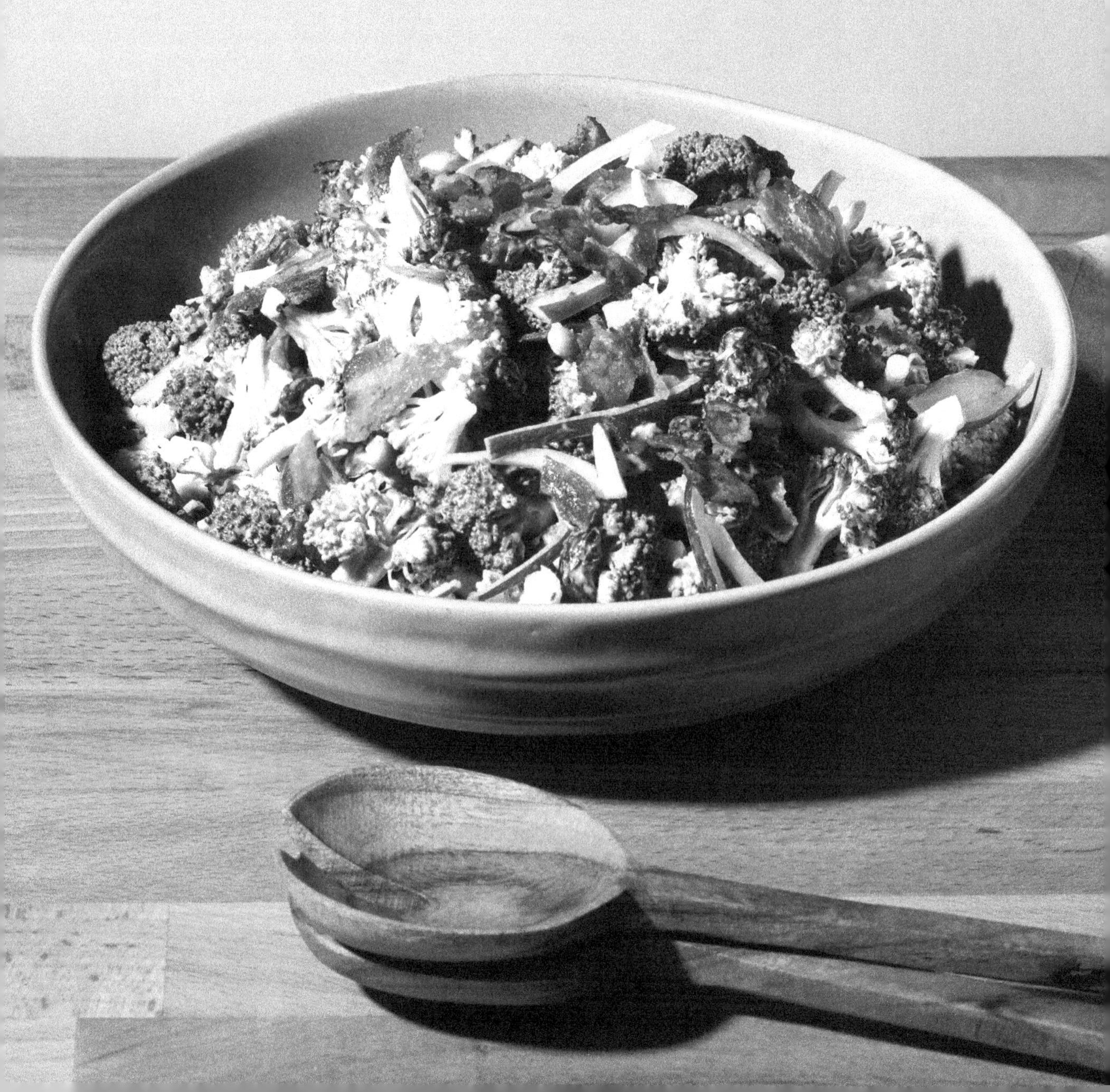

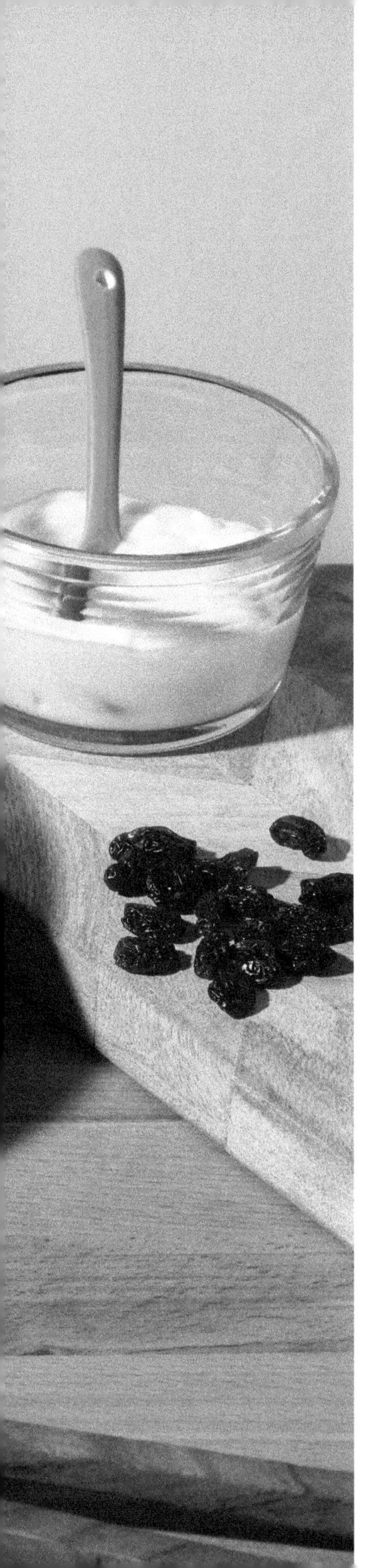

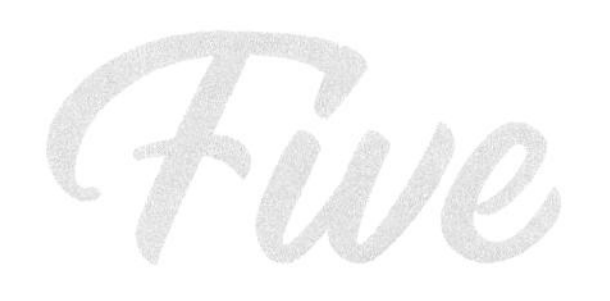

# Five

# Salads and Soups

# CUCUMBER, TOMATO, AND RED ONION SALAD

**Serves 4**
**Prep time: 10 minutes**

*Egg-Free, Gluten-Free, Nut-Free, Soy-Free, Vegan*

When you need to make a dish ahead of time, this is a perfect option. This salad actually gets better as it sits in the dressing in the fridge for a few hours (or up to a few days), as it absorbs the flavor. The sugar added to the dressing helps tame the acidity of the vinegar and any bitterness in the cucumber.

- 4 medium tomatoes, quartered and cut into ¼-inch-thick slices
- 2 cucumbers, peeled and cut into ¼-inch-thick rounds
- ¼ red onion, sliced
- 2 tablespoons extra-virgin olive oil
- 2 tablespoons distilled white vinegar
- 1 tablespoon sugar
- ½ teaspoon salt

In a large bowl, combine the tomatoes, cucumbers, and red onion.

In a small bowl, whisk together the oil, vinegar, sugar, and salt. Pour over the tomato and cucumber mixture and toss everything well to combine.

Serve immediately, or store covered in the refrigerator for up to 4 days.

*Mix it up:* Try different types of vinegar in this recipe for slight taste variations. I also love using red wine vinegar or balsamic vinegar.

---

**Per Serving:** Calories: 106; Total fat: 7g; Carbohydrates: 10g; Cholesterol: 0mg; Fiber: 2g; Protein: 1g; Sugar: 8g

# MANGO AVOCADO SALAD

**Serves 4**

**Prep time: 10 minutes**

*Egg-Free, Gluten-Free, Nut-Free, Soy-Free, Vegan*

This simple side dish pairs wonderfully with grilled steak, roasted chicken, or fish tacos. You can also mix this salad with cooked rice and a can of black, pinto, or small white beans for a quick Meatless Monday meal. Since avocado browns quickly, I recommend making this dish right before you plan to eat it so the avocado retains its bright green color.

2 mangos, chopped
2 avocados, chopped
1 tablespoon extra-virgin olive oil
Juice of ½ lime
2 tablespoons chopped fresh cilantro
⅛ teaspoon salt

In a medium bowl, toss together all the ingredients. Serve immediately.

*Substitution tip:* You can also prepare this with pineapple (2 cups fresh or canned) instead of mango. If you find it too sweet this way, add a little sliced red onion, which nicely counters the sweet pineapple and rich avocado.

---

**Per Serving:** Calories: 244; Total fat: 14g; Carbohydrates: 31g; Cholesterol: 0mg; Fiber: 7.5g; Protein: 3g; Sugar: 23g

# CRUNCHY BROCCOLI SALAD

**Serves 6**
**Prep time: 15 minutes / Cook time: 10 minutes**

Whether you need to bring food to a potluck barbecue or want a new veggie to serve at a family dinner, this crunchy broccoli salad will become your go-to choice. The side dish comes together quickly, since only the bacon requires cooking–it's a great use for leftover cooked bacon. I find the crisp raw broccoli adds a refreshing crunch. Since it's uncooked, though, be sure to cut the florets into small pieces.

5 bacon slices
2 heads broccoli, chopped into small florets (about 1 pound of florets)
⅓ cup chopped red onion
¾ cup golden raisins
¾ cup mayonnaise
1½ tablespoons distilled white vinegar
3 tablespoons sugar

In a large skillet, cook the bacon until crisp. Set the bacon aside on paper towels until cool, then crumble into small pieces.

In a large bowl, combine the broccoli, red onion, and raisins.

In a small bowl, combine the mayonnaise, vinegar, and sugar. Pour the dressing over the broccoli and toss well, until fully coated.

Add the bacon and serve immediately, or store covered in the refrigerator for up to 4 days. If saving for another day, store the bacon separately until ready to serve. Toss everything again right before serving, as the dressing may settle at the bottom of the bowl.

*Protein swap:* Instead of bacon, add ⅓ cup roasted sunflower seeds, tossing them in at the last minute so they stay crisp. Make that change along with swapping out the mayonnaise for a vegan mayo, and you've made the whole dish vegan.

---

**Per Serving:** Calories: 344; Total fat: 24g; Carbohydrates: 28g; Cholesterol: 21mg; Fiber: 2.5g; Protein: 7g; Sugar: 20g

# BUFFALO CHICKPEA SALAD

**Serves 4**
**Prep time: 15 minutes / Cook time: 5 minutes**

*Gluten-Free, Nut-Free, Vegetarian*

Get a little spicy with this salad! Fiber-rich chickpeas are lightly toasted on the stovetop, then covered in hot sauce. By combining the chickpeas with bitter red onion, rich avocado, and creamy ranch dressing, you'll treat your taste buds to a wonderful blend of flavors using minimal ingredients.

3 tablespoons olive oil, divided
1 (15.5-ounce) can chickpeas, rinsed and drained
2½ tablespoons hot sauce
8 to 10 ounces green leaf lettuce, coarsely chopped
¼ red onion, sliced
2 avocados, chopped
8 tablespoons Ranch Dressing (page 39)

1. In a large skillet, heat 1½ tablespoons of olive oil over medium heat. Add the chickpeas and cook, stirring occasionally, for 4 minutes. Stir in the remaining 1½ tablespoons of olive oil and the hot sauce, cooking for an additional minute, until everything is well combined.
2. Divide the lettuce evenly among four plates and top with the chickpeas. Add red onion and avocado to each plate, then top with the ranch dressing.

*Protein swap:* To make this a meat-based meal, swap out the chickpeas for 1 pound of chicken. You can cut up the chicken and cook it in the oil in the skillet in step 1. Simply increase the cooking time to 8 to 10 minutes, or until the chicken is fully cooked, before tossing in the hot sauce.

---

**Per Serving:** Calories: 441; Total fat: 36g; Carbohydrates: 25g; Cholesterol: 8mg; Fiber: 10g; Protein: 7g; Sugar: 4g

# BLT PASTA SALAD

**Serves 4**
**Prep time: 20 minutes / Cook time: 20 minutes**

If you enjoy a classic BLT sandwich, you'll love this recipe, which is perfect for a summertime get-together, but also filling enough for a quick dinner. It's best made and served warm. When stored in the fridge, the pasta has a tendency to soak up some of the dressing and it can dry out a bit. You can fix this by adding a little extra mayonnaise and oat milk to the leftovers and tossing everything prior to serving.

6 ounces farfalle pasta
6 bacon slices
1 pint cherry tomatoes, halved
5 to 6 ounces green leaf lettuce, chopped
⅓ cup mayonnaise
2 tablespoons unsweetened oat milk or other dairy-free milk
¼ teaspoon salt
¼ teaspoon freshly ground black pepper
¼ teaspoon dried minced garlic
¼ teaspoon red pepper flakes

Cook the pasta according to package directions. Drain and set the pasta aside in a large bowl.

Meanwhile, in a large skillet, cook the bacon until crisp. Transfer to paper towels to cool. Crumble and add it to the bowl with the pasta.

Add the tomatoes and lettuce to the bowl.

In a small bowl, combine the mayonnaise, oat milk, salt, black pepper, garlic, and pepper flakes. Whisk well.

Pour the dressing over the pasta salad. Toss everything well to combine and serve.

*Mix it up:* Jazz this up however you wish. You can add chopped avocado or bell pepper, or swap out the lettuce for baby spinach.

---

**Per Serving:** Calories: 371; Total fat: 19g; Carbohydrates: 37g; Cholesterol: 19mg; Fiber: 3.5g; Protein: 12g; Sugar: 3.5g

# ROASTED POTATO AND ARUGULA SALAD

**Serves 4**
**Prep time: 15 minutes / Cook time: 35 minutes**

*Egg-Free, Gluten-Free, Soy-Free, Vegetarian*

This is a wonderful warm salad to include on your wintertime menu. Seasoned potatoes combined with peppery arugula and a bright lemon dressing, all topped off with Dairy-Free Parmesan, makes for a simple, delectable salad that everyone will love.

1½ pounds Yukon Gold or other potatoes, cut into 1-inch pieces
2 tablespoons olive oil
½ teaspoon salt
½ teaspoon garlic powder
½ teaspoon paprika
¼ teaspoon freshly ground black pepper
5 ounces baby arugula
4 tablespoons Dairy-Free Parmesan (page 36)
Lemon Vinaigrette Dressing (page 76)

1. Preheat the oven to 425°F.
2. On a baking sheet, toss the potatoes with the olive oil, salt, garlic powder, paprika, and pepper. Bake for 35 to 45 minutes, stirring once halfway through, until the potatoes are lightly crisp on the outside and tender on the inside.
3. Serve the potatoes over the arugula. Top with the Parmesan and lemon vinaigrette.

*Make it easier:* Use a store-bought vinaigrette dressing and dairy-free Parmesan. Though the Parmesan may not be stocked at all supermarkets, natural foods stores often carry this item.

---

**Per Serving:** Calories: 385; Total fat: 24g; Carbohydrates: 41g; Cholesterol: 0mg; Fiber: 4g; Protein: 5g; Sugar: 12g

# HONEY-MUSTARD POTATO SALAD

**Serves 6**

**Prep time: 15 minutes / Cook time: 40 minutes**

Put a new spin on potato salad with this recipe, which switches out traditional mayonnaise dressing for a homemade honey-mustard version. This salad is best served warm rather than cold, but if you want to make it ahead of time, roast the potatoes and prepare the dressing, but keep them separate. When ready to serve, reheat the potatoes in the oven until warm and crisp and then toss them in the dressing.

- 2 pounds russet potatoes, cut into bite-size chunks
- 4 tablespoons olive oil, divided
- ½ teaspoon salt
- 2 tablespoons honey
- 2 tablespoons grainy mustard
- 1 tablespoon apple cider vinegar
- ¼ cup chopped fresh parsley

Preheat the oven to 400°F.

Place the potatoes on a baking sheet. Drizzle with 2 tablespoons of oil and sprinkle with the salt, then toss to evenly coat. Bake for 40 to 45 minutes, or until the potatoes are tender inside and crisp outside, stirring once halfway through.

Meanwhile, in a small bowl, whisk together the honey, mustard, vinegar, and remaining 2 tablespoons of olive oil.

Toss the warm roasted potatoes in a large bowl with the dressing and chopped parsley. Serve immediately.

*Protein swap:* For a quick dinner, toss some precooked chicken into this potato salad, and you've got a complete main course.

---

**Per Serving:** Calories: 200; Total fat: 9g; Carbohydrates: 26g; Cholesterol: 0mg; Fiber: 3g; Protein: 3g; Sugar: 1.5g

# ROASTED VEGETABLE SALAD

**Serves 4**

**Prep time: 20 minutes / Cook time: 30 minutes**

*Egg-Free, Nut-Free, Soy-Free Option, Vegetarian*

When I travel for work, I sometimes end up eating less-nutritious choices. When I return home, this salad is always the first thing I make to reset into healthy habits. Loaded with different vegetables, this medley provides fiber along with a wide variety of vitamins and minerals. Though I use my standard Lemon Vinaigrette Dressing here, feel free to swap in another dressing of your choice.

1 pint cherry tomatoes
1 large zucchini, cut into ½-inch-thick rounds
4 tablespoons olive oil, divided
1 red onion, quartered, then separated layer by layer
1 red bell pepper, cut into strips
1 small eggplant, peeled and cut into 1-inch cubes
1 teaspoon salt
4 ounces Italian bread (½ small loaf, soy-free if needed), halved lengthwise
8 ounces green leaf lettuce
Lemon Vinaigrette Dressing (page 76)

1. Preheat the oven to 400°F.
2. Place the cherry tomatoes and zucchini on a baking sheet and drizzle with 1 tablespoon of oil. Place the red onion, bell pepper, and eggplant on another baking sheet and drizzle with 2 tablespoons of oil. Sprinkle the salt evenly over all the vegetables. Stir the vegetables to fully coat them, then place both pans in the oven.
3. Bake the pan with the tomatoes and zucchini for 15 to 20 minutes, or until the zucchini is fork tender. Leave the other pan in for an additional 5 to 10 minutes (around 25 minutes total), or until the vegetables are fork tender and appear a little charred around the edges.
4. Brush the soft part of the bread with the remaining 1 tablespoon of oil. Place the bread on a baking sheet, oiled-side up, and bake for 5 minutes, or until crisp. Remove from the oven and cut into bite-size pieces.

Top the lettuce with the roasted vegetables and chopped bread. Toss with the lemon vinaigrette.

*Protein swap:* This is a hearty salad as is, but you can also add roasted chicken or grilled shrimp for more protein. You can likely get 6 servings out of this with the addition of meat or fish; just add a little more lettuce if needed.

*Mix it up:* In the summertime, grill the vegetables and bread rather than roasting them in the oven.

---

**Per Serving:** Calories: 426; Total fat: 29g; Carbohydrates: 40g; Cholesterol: 0mg; Fiber: 6g; Protein: 6g; Sugar: 19g

# BARBECUE BEEF SALAD

**Serves 4**
**Prep time: 15 minutes / Cook time: 10 minutes**

*Nut-Free, Gluten-Free Option*

When my husband and I started dating, I remember him (half) joking when he told me "salads are for sides, not for meals." I like to think I've changed his mind with this barbecue beef salad. It's the best dish to bridge the gap between the salad lovers and the meat-and-potatoes crowd. I use my homemade dairy-free Ranch Dressing combined with barbecue sauce for the dressing, but you can easily swap that out for a store-bought dressing to save time.

1 pound ground beef (90% lean)
½ small red onion, chopped
½ cup barbecue sauce, plus 3 tablespoons (certified gluten-free if needed), divided
8 to 10 ounces romaine lettuce, chopped
1 cup canned corn kernels, drained
1 (15.5-ounce) can black beans, rinsed and drained
1½ cups cherry tomatoes, halved
6 tablespoons Ranch Dressing (page 39)
10 to 15 corn tortilla chips, crushed (optional)

1. In a large skillet, cook the ground beef and red onion over medium heat, stirring frequently and breaking up the meat, for 7 to 10 minutes, or until the beef is browned. Drain any excess fat, then stir in ½ cup of barbecue sauce. Remove from the heat.
2. Divide the lettuce among four plates. Top with the beef, corn, black beans, and tomatoes.
3. In a small bowl, stir together the ranch dressing and remaining 3 tablespoons of barbecue sauce. Use this to dress the salad. If desired, sprinkle crushed tortilla chips over the top of the salad.

*Protein swap:* Substitute ground turkey or chicken for the ground beef, or even some vegan meat crumbles, which are typically soy-based.

---

**Per Serving:** Calories: 255; Total fat: 9g; Carbohydrates: 30g; Cholesterol: 76mg; Fiber: 6g; Protein: 14g; Sugar: 24g

# CUCUMBER AND MANGO GAZPACHO

**Serves 4**

**Prep time: 15 minutes, plus 1 hour to chill**

*Egg-Free, Gluten-Free, Nut-Free, Soy-Free, Vegan*

Soup isn't just for winter; you can enjoy it all summer long with this refreshing gazpacho—in fact, this soup, rooted in Spanish cuisine and traditionally made with a tomato base and other blended vegetables, is always served cold. This version takes an untraditional route by swapping the tomatoes for a cucumber and mango base. You don't even need to cook anything; just blend, chill, and eat!

1 English cucumber, peeled and coarsely chopped
2 mangos, coarsely chopped
½ bell pepper (any color), coarsely chopped
1 jalapeño pepper, seeded
¼ cup fresh cilantro leaves
3 tablespoons extra-virgin olive oil
Juice of 1 lime
½ teaspoon salt

In a large high-powered blender, combine the cucumber, mangos, bell pepper, jalapeño, cilantro, oil, lime juice, and salt and blend for 1 to 2 minutes. Place the blender jar in the refrigerator for 1 hour, or until chilled.

When ready to serve, either eat as is or, for a smoother texture, pour through a fine-mesh sieve into a bowl. You may need to frequently stir the mixture as it sits in the sieve in order to help push the liquid through to the bowl (discard any pulp in the sieve). Serve the smooth gazpacho.

*Mix it up:* Gazpacho can be made from any variety of vegetables and fruits. Try a watermelon and cucumber gazpacho, using mint leaves rather than cilantro, or a traditional tomato gazpacho, which is especially delicious with fresh summer tomatoes.

---

**Per Serving:** Calories: 208; Total fat: 11g; Carbohydrates: 29g; Cholesterol: 0mg; Fiber: 4g; Protein: 2g; Sugar: 25g

# CREAMY TOMATO SOUP

**Serves 4**
**Prep time: 15 minutes / Cook time: 35 minutes**

*Egg-Free, Gluten-Free, Nut-Free, Soy-Free*

A local farm near where I live offers an amazing discount on heirloom tomatoes each summer. I try to swing by every year, and stock up on the gorgeous yellow, red, orange, and plum-colored tomatoes, all in unique shapes and sizes. Combined, they provide extraordinary fresh flavor in this creamy tomato soup. Of course, if you don't have heirloom varieties available by you, standard tomatoes will do the job well, too.

4 bacon slices, chopped into bite-size pieces
1 yellow onion, chopped
2 garlic cloves, minced
6 cups chopped heirloom tomatoes
1 large potato, peeled and chopped
2 cups chicken broth
1 teaspoon Italian seasoning
¼ teaspoon salt

1. In a large pot, cook the bacon over medium heat, stirring occasionally, until crisp. Remove it with a slotted spoon and set aside, leaving the bacon grease in the pot.
2. Add the onion to the pot and cook over medium heat, stirring occasionally, for 3 to 4 minutes, or until the onion starts to become tender. Add the garlic and cook, stirring, for another minute.
3. Add the tomatoes, potato, broth, Italian seasoning, and salt. Reduce the heat to low and simmer for 20 to 30 minutes, or until the potatoes are tender.
4. Purée the soup with an immersion blender, then ladle into bowls and top with the reserved bacon.

*Make it easier:* If you don't have an immersion blender, just wait for the soup to cool down, then use a regular blender to carefully purée, working in batches. Cover the top with a towel to prevent spattering. Pour it back into the pot and set over medium heat for a minute or two until warm, for serving.

---

**Per Serving:** Calories: 186; Total fat: 12g; Carbohydrates: 14g; Cholesterol: 21mg; Fiber: 3.5g; Protein: 7g; Sugar: 9g

# PUMPKIN AND APPLE SOUP

**Serves 4**

**Prep time: 10 minutes / Cook time: 20 minutes**

*Egg-Free, Gluten-Free, Nut-Free, Soy-Free, Vegan*

Embrace the fall season with this cozy pumpkin soup. It delivers the perfect blend of sweetness from the pumpkin and apple, savory elements from the onion and broth, and richness from the coconut milk. Serve it alongside a salad or fresh baked bread for a light and filling lunch or dinner. Bonus: This soup takes only 30 minutes to prepare, from start to finish!

1 tablespoon olive oil
1 medium yellow onion, chopped
2 garlic cloves, minced
1 small apple, peeled and chopped
1 teaspoon curry powder
¼ teaspoon salt
¼ teaspoon freshly ground black pepper
1 (15-ounce) can unsweetened pumpkin purée
2 cups vegetable broth
1 cup canned full-fat coconut milk, plus a drizzle for serving
Pumpkin seeds (optional)

In a medium pot, heat the oil over medium heat. Add the onion and cook for 3 to 4 minutes, stirring occasionally, until it starts to become tender. Add the garlic and cook, stirring, for another minute. Add the apple, curry powder, salt, and pepper. Cook for 2 to 3 minutes.

Stir in the pumpkin purée and broth. Simmer for 10 minutes over low heat.

Pour in the coconut milk and remove from the heat. Use an immersion blender to purée the soup, then ladle into bowls. Garnish with another drizzle of coconut milk and pumpkin seeds (if using).

*Substitution tip:* To make this with butternut squash instead of pumpkin, add 1½ pounds of peeled, cubed butternut to the recipe in the first step. In the second step, omit the pumpkin purée and add 3 cups of broth. Let the squash simmer in the broth until tender. Proceed as directed.

---

**Per Serving:** Calories: 232; Total fat: 17g; Carbohydrates: 20g; Cholesterol: 0mg; Fiber: 5g; Protein: 2.5g; Sugar: 10g

# CORN CHOWDER

**Serves 6**

**Prep time: 20 minutes, plus overnight to soak / Cook time: 35 minutes**

*Egg-Free, Soy-Free, Vegan Option (see tip)*

Corn chowder is one of my favorite summer dishes, but this recipe uses canned corn, for year-round versatility. Don't skip the cashew cream, as it adds a rich, creamy thickness to the soup.

½ cup raw cashews
6 bacon slices, cut into bite-size pieces
1 small onion, chopped
1 bell pepper (any color), chopped
1 garlic clove, minced
2 tablespoons all-purpose flour
3½ cups chicken broth, divided
1 pound Yukon Gold or other potatoes, peeled and chopped
½ teaspoon salt
¼ teaspoon freshly ground black pepper
2 (15-ounce) cans corn kernels, undrained

1. Put the cashews in a mason jar and add enough water to cover the nuts by a few inches. Soak in the refrigerator for at least 8 and up to 24 hours. Drain and rinse the cashews.
2. In a large pot, cook the bacon over medium heat, stirring occasionally, until crisp. Remove with a slotted spoon and set aside, leaving the bacon grease in the pot.
3. Add the onion and bell pepper to the pot and cook over medium heat for 5 to 7 minutes, or until the bell pepper starts to get tender. Add the garlic and cook, stirring, for another minute. Add the flour, stirring to coat the vegetables. Slowly mix in 3 cups of chicken broth, then add the potatoes, salt, and black pepper. Bring to a boil and cook for about 10 minutes, or until the potatoes are tender.
4. Meanwhile, add the cashews to a food processer or high-powered blender. Process in 30-second increments, stirring as necessary, until a thick paste forms. Add the remaining ½ cup of broth and pulse until the mixture is creamy.
5. Add the corn with its liquid to the pot, along with the cashew cream. Cook for 5 minutes. Use an immersion blender to blend about half the soup, so some remains chunky. Portion into bowls and top with the bacon.

*Mix it up:* To make this vegan, skip the bacon, use olive oil to sauté the vegetables, and sub vegetable broth for the chicken broth.

---

**Per Serving:** Calories: 319; Total fat: 17g; Carbohydrates: 34g; Cholesterol: 18mg; Fiber: 5.5g; Protein: 9g; Sugar: 11g

# LEMONY WHITE BEAN AND ORZO SOUP

**Serves 4**

**Prep time: 10 minutes / Cook time: 20 minutes**

*Egg-Free, Nut-Free, Soy-Free, Vegan Option (see tip)*

The warm broth and bright pop of lemon make this soup a welcome treat on a cold winter day. This dish comes together in just under 30 minutes, perfect for a quick weeknight meal. You'll also find this a soothing option when you or your kiddos feel under the weather; it's a nice alternative to chicken noodle soup.

1 tablespoon olive oil
1 small yellow onion, chopped
2 garlic cloves, minced
¼ cup white wine
4 cups chicken broth
2 thyme sprigs
1 rosemary sprig
1 bay leaf
¾ cup orzo
Juice of 1 lemon
1 (15-ounce) can white beans, rinsed and drained
2 cups packed baby spinach

In a large pot, heat the olive oil over medium heat. Add the onion and garlic and cook, stirring frequently, for 5 minutes, or until softened. Pour in the wine and let everything cook for another 1 to 2 minutes.

Add the broth, thyme, rosemary, and bay leaf. Increase the heat and bring to a boil. Add the orzo and reduce the heat to medium-low, letting the mixture simmer for 8 minutes.

Stir in the lemon juice, beans, and spinach and cook for an additional 2 minutes, or until the spinach is wilted and the orzo is tender. Discard the rosemary, thyme, and bay leaf. Serve immediately.

*Substitution tip:* Swap out the chicken broth for vegetable broth to make this a vegan meal. Feel free to make other substitutions based on what you've got on hand in your kitchen. Small pasta shapes can be used in place of orzo, or kale can be swapped in for spinach.

---

**Per Serving:** Calories: 268; Total fat: 4.5g; Carbohydrates: 43g; Cholesterol: 5mg; Fiber: 7g; Protein: 13g; Sugar: 5g

# RED CURRY CHICKEN AND ZOODLE SOUP

**Serves 4**
**Prep time: 15 minutes / Cook time: 20 minutes**

*Egg-Free, Gluten-Free, Nut-Free*

Curry is a comfort food for me, so I turn to this red curry chicken and zoodle soup during stressful times. Spiralized zucchini adds a noodle-esque quality to the meal. If you don't own a spiralizer, simply run a peeler over your zucchini repeatedly, forming pappardelle-style noodles for your soup.

- 1 tablespoon olive oil
- 1 pound boneless, skinless chicken breast, cut into bite-size pieces
- ¼ teaspoon salt
- ½ yellow onion, chopped
- 2 tablespoons red curry paste
- 1 (14.5-ounce) can diced tomatoes, undrained
- 2 cups chicken broth
- 1 (15-ounce) can full-fat coconut milk
- Juice of 1 lime
- ¼ cup chopped fresh cilantro
- 2 zucchini, peeled and spiralized

1. In a large pot, heat the olive oil over medium heat. Season the chicken breast with the salt, then add to the pot. Add the onion and cook for 8 to 10 minutes, stirring every few minutes, until the chicken is cooked through.
2. Stir in the curry paste and cook for an additional minute. Add the tomatoes with their juices and the chicken broth and bring to a boil. Reduce the heat to medium-low and let simmer for 5 minutes.
3. Add the coconut milk, lime juice, cilantro, and zucchini and cook for 2 to 4 minutes, or until the zucchini is crisp-tender.

*Make it easier:* Shave off a few minutes by using leftover cooked chicken, rather than cooking the chicken in step 1.

---

**Per Serving:** Calories: 441; Total fat: 30g; Carbohydrates: 15g; Cholesterol: 85mg; Fiber: 4g; Protein: 31g; Sugar: 7g

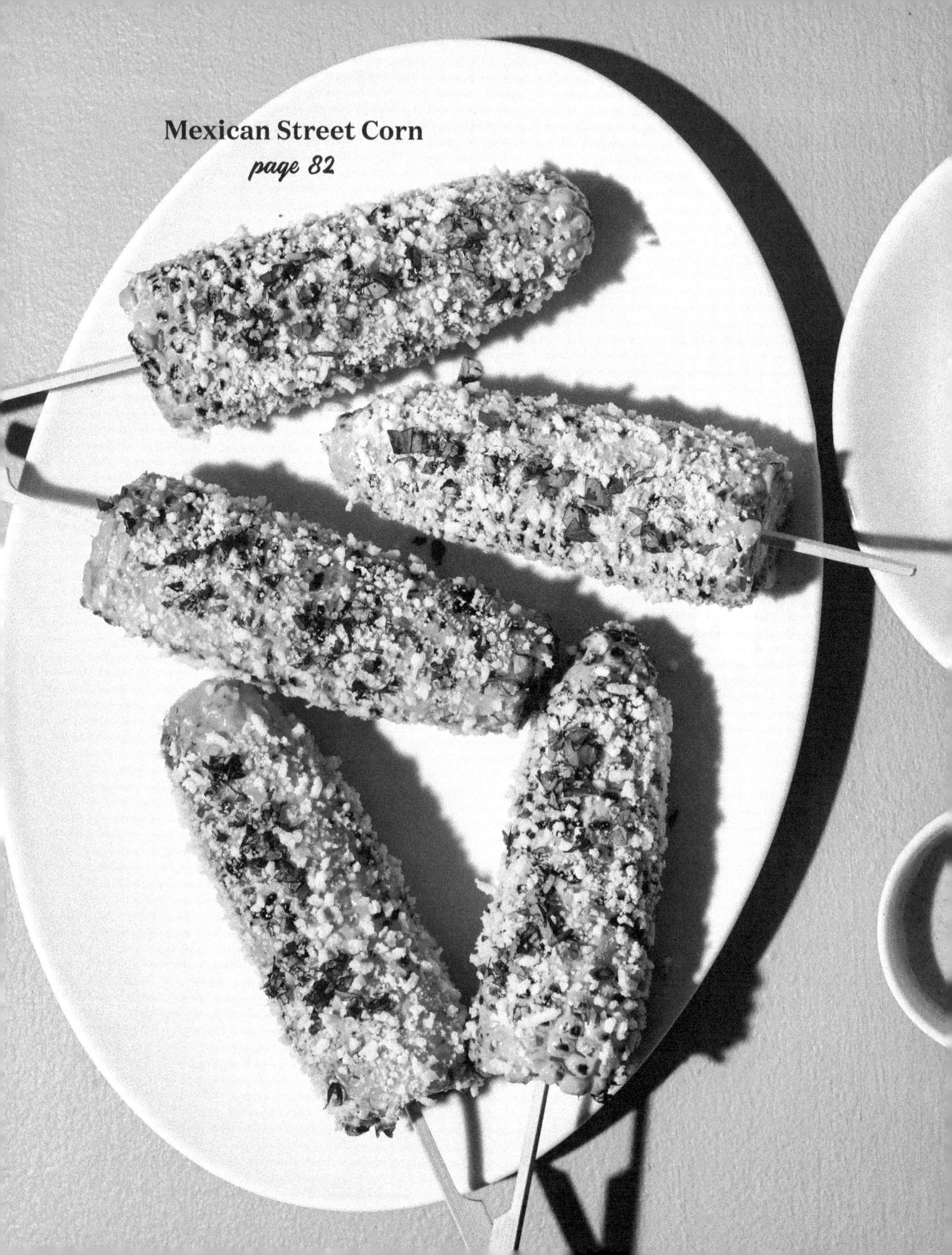

Mexican Street Corn
*page 82*

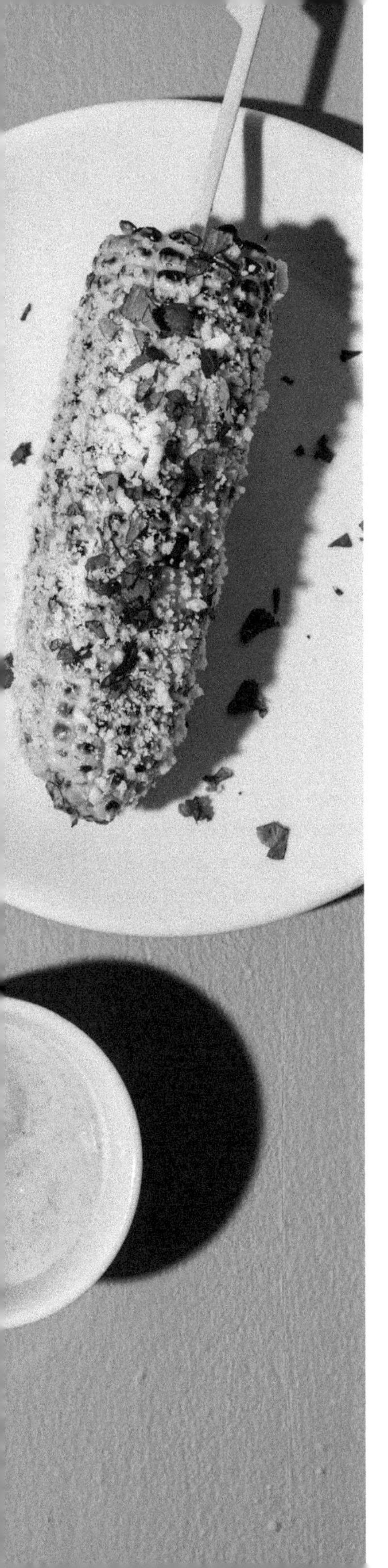

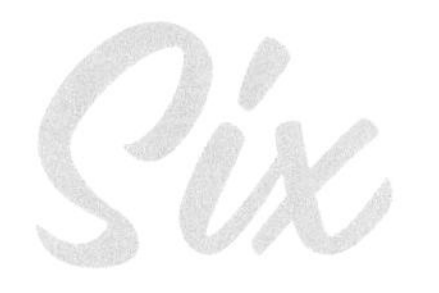

# Six

# Sauces, Sides, and Snacks

# LEMON VINAIGRETTE DRESSING

**Makes ½ cup**
**Prep time: 10 minutes**

When you have a few basic dressing recipes on hand, like dairy-free Ranch Dressing (page 39) and this vibrant lemon vinaigrette, you'll always be ready to make delicious salads. Traditional vinaigrette recipes call for a ratio of 3:1 oil to acid (vinegar or citrus juice). For this recipe, though, I prefer a blend of half oil and half lemon juice for a citrus-forward vinaigrette that's lightly sweetened with honey. Use it for drizzling on salads or marinating chicken.

¼ cup fresh lemon juice
¼ cup extra-virgin olive oil
2 tablespoons honey
1 teaspoon minced garlic
¼ teaspoon salt
⅛ teaspoon freshly ground black pepper

In a screw-top jar, combine the lemon juice, olive oil, honey, garlic, salt, and pepper. Close the lid and shake to combine well. Serve immediately. Store leftovers in the refrigerator for up to 5 days. The oil may separate in the refrigerator; leave at room temperature for 15 minutes and shake well before serving.

*Mix it up:* Get creative! You can swap out lemon juice for lime juice, and add a little cilantro. Or try combining equal parts orange juice and olive oil, then mixing in a little mayo, lemon juice, and sugar for a creamy citrus dressing.

---

**Per Serving (2 tablespoons):** Calories: 156; Total fat: 14g; Carbohydrates: 10g; Cholesterol: 0mg; Fiber: 0g; Protein: 0g; Sugar: 9g

# MUSHROOM AND SWEET ONION GRAVY

**Serves 4**

**Prep time: 10 minutes / Cook time: 10 minutes**

*Egg-Free, Nut-Free, Soy-Free, Vegan Option*

You're probably familiar with the four basic tastes of sweet, salty, sour, and bitter. But did you know there's a fifth recognized taste called *umami*? Umami is a savory perception, and in this recipe it's found specifically in the mushrooms. The saltiness of the vegan butter and chicken broth, and the sweetness in the sautéed onions, make this gravy a delicious addition to your table. Serve over turkey, chicken, Creamy Mashed Potatoes (page 83), or rice.

- 4 tablespoons vegan butter or olive oil
- ½ cup chopped sweet onion
- 1 cup chopped baby bella (cremini) mushrooms
- ¼ cup all-purpose flour
- 2 cups chicken broth (or vegetable broth for vegan option)
- ¼ teaspoon salt
- ¼ teaspoon freshly ground black pepper

1. In a large sauté pan, melt the butter over medium heat. Add the onion and mushrooms and cook, stirring occasionally, for 5 to 7 minutes, or until the vegetables are tender.
2. Stir in the flour. Let cook for about 30 seconds and then slowly add the chicken broth while constantly stirring.
3. Add the salt and pepper and let the gravy cook for another minute. Remove from the heat and serve immediately.

*Mix it up:* If you've just roasted a chicken or turkey, you can use the pan drippings to add extra flavor to this recipe. Use just 1 tablespoon of vegan butter to sauté your vegetables and then add about ¼ cup of drippings to the pan. Proceed as directed.

**Per Serving:** Calories: 148; Total fat: 11g; Carbohydrates: 9g; Cholesterol: 2mg; Fiber: 0.5g; Protein: 2g; Sugar: 2g

# QUICK-PICKLED RED ONIONS

**Makes about 1½ cups**

**Prep time: 5 minutes, plus 15 minutes rest time / Cook time: 5 minutes**

*Egg-Free, Gluten-Free, Nut-Free, Soy-Free, Vegetarian*

Once you try these pickled red onions, you'll always want to keep them on hand. The bitter onions are transformed into a salty-sweet delight via a quick-pickling process and can be used to add a pop of flavor in dishes like tacos and salads. To avoid spilling the hot vinegar on your hands or counters, put the jar of onions in an empty sink to catch any spills as you pour.

1 large red onion, thinly sliced
½ cup distilled white vinegar
½ cup water
2 tablespoons honey
1 teaspoon salt

1. Put the sliced red onion in a 1-pint mason jar, packing in the onion toward the bottom of the jar as much as possible.
2. In a medium pot, combine the vinegar, water, honey, and salt and bring to a boil over medium heat. Remove from the heat and carefully pour the mixture into the jar with the onion.
3. Let the jar with the onion sit at room temperature for 15 to 20 minutes. Use immediately, or store in the refrigerator for up to 1 week.

*Mix it up:* You can use this quick-pickling technique with other vegetables, like carrots, cauliflower, and cucumbers. For these, you might wish to add other seasonings to the jar, like peppercorns, dill, and/or garlic.

---

**Per Serving (¼ cup):** Calories: 31; Total fat: 0g; Carbohydrates: 8g; Cholesterol: 0mg; Fiber: 0.5g; Protein: 0g; Sugar: 7g

# BALSAMIC HONEY COLLARD GREENS

**Serves 4**
**Prep time: 10 minutes / Cook time: 30 minutes**

*Egg-Free, Nut-Free, Soy-Free, Gluten-Free*

Collard greens are a soul-food staple packed with beta-carotene and vitamin C. Some of the very best collard greens I've had have been when I visited family in the South, where they are traditionally simmered for hours and accentuated with salty, smoked ham. But you can cook collards in many different ways. It's fun to experiment with unique flavor combinations, like this balsamic honey version. Try serving alongside grilled or Fried Chicken (page 130).

1 bunch collard greens (1½ to 2 pounds)
1 tablespoon olive oil
½ yellow onion, chopped
1 cup chicken broth
2 tablespoons balsamic vinegar
1 tablespoon honey
¼ teaspoon salt
⅛ teaspoon freshly ground black pepper

1. Fold each collard green leaf in half lengthwise and cut out the tough midrib from the center (discard the midribs and stems). Chop the leaves.
2. In a large sauté pan or skillet, heat the oil over medium heat. Add the onion and cook, stirring occasionally, for 4 to 5 minutes, or until the onion starts to get tender.
3. Add the collard greens and chicken broth. Bring to a boil, then reduce the heat to simmer, cover, and cook for 15 to 20 minutes, or until the collards are tender.
4. Stir in the vinegar, honey, salt, and pepper. Continue to cook uncovered for another 5 minutes to blend the flavors, then serve.

*Mix it up:* In addition to cooking collard greens as a side dish, try them as a wrap for sandwiches, cooked in a stir-fry, or added to an omelet.

---

**Per Serving:** Calories: 138; Total fat: 5g; Carbohydrates: 20g; Cholesterol: 1mg; Fiber: 9.5g; Protein: 7g; Sugar: 7g

# BACON-WRAPPED GREEN BEANS

**Serves 8**
**Prep time: 15 minutes / Cook time: 30 minutes**

This recipe was the only way my mom could get me to eat green beans when I was a kid. As an adult, I've expanded my palate considerably, but this is still one of my favorite ways to prepare them. Bacon-wrapped green beans make an indulgent side dish or appetizer for a holiday party. Some people blanch the green beans and partially cook the bacon ahead of time, but I find that wrapping everything raw and cooking for a little longer leads to the same great texture and taste. As the bacon renders in the oven, the grease helps cook the beans inside.

80 green beans (about 2 pounds), ends trimmed
16 bacon slices (about 1 pound)
2 tablespoons brown sugar

Preheat the oven to 375°F.

Take 5 green beans and wrap them in a slice of bacon, starting toward the top of the bundle and wrapping your way around toward the bottom. Place the bundle on a baking sheet. Repeat with the remaining green beans and bacon. Sprinkle the bundles with the brown sugar.

Bake for 30 to 40 minutes, or until the bacon is cooked through and the green beans are tender. Serve hot. Store leftovers in the refrigerator for up to 4 days.

*Ingredient tip:* If you're trying to reduce sugar in your diet, feel free to leave the brown sugar out of this recipe.

---

**Per Serving (2 bundles):** Calories: 138; Total fat: 8g; Carbohydrates: 8g; Cholesterol: 23mg; Fiber: 1.5g; Protein: 9g; Sugar: 5g

# MAPLE-MUSTARD ROASTED CARROTS

**Serves 4**
**Prep time: 10 minutes / Cook time: 35 minutes**

*Egg-Free, Gluten-Free, Nut-Free, Soy-Free, Vegan*

Carrots are an excellent source of beta-carotene, the plant pigment that gives this veggie its bright orange color. Studies have shown that diets rich in carotenoids (like beta-carotene) are associated with reduced risk of diseases like cancer and cardiovascular disease. Roasting carrots brings out their sweetness, and tossing them in a simple maple-mustard glaze adds even more depth of flavor.

1 pound baby carrots, halved lengthwise
1½ tablespoons olive oil
¼ teaspoon salt
1 tablespoon pure maple syrup
1 tablespoon grainy mustard

1. Preheat the oven to 425°F.
2. Place the carrots on a baking sheet. Drizzle with the oil and sprinkle with the salt, tossing the carrots to evenly coat.
3. Bake for 35 to 40 minutes, stirring once halfway through, until the carrots are tender and have started to caramelize.
4. In a medium bowl, combine the maple syrup and mustard. Add the roasted carrots to the bowl and toss well to coat in the maple-mustard glaze. Serve immediately. Store leftovers in the refrigerator for up to 4 days.

*Substitution tip:* Swap out the maple syrup for honey (though it won't be vegan) or the grainy mustard for Dijon or spicy mustard, depending on what you have on hand.

---

**Per Serving:** Calories: 101; Total fat: 5g; Carbohydrates: 13g; Cholesterol: 0mg; Fiber: 3g; Protein: 1g; Sugar: 8.5g

# MEXICAN STREET CORN

**Serves 6**

**Prep time: 10 minutes / Cook time: 10 minutes**

Mix things up with this summertime staple by swapping your usual buttered corn for *elotes*, or Mexican street corn. This snack or side dish is traditionally coated in mayonnaise or *crema*, chili powder, cilantro, and lime, then topped with Cotija cheese or queso fresco. To make it dairy-free, we'll stick with a mayonnaise mixture and top it off with Dairy-Free Parmesan.

6 ears corn, husked
½ cup mayonnaise
Juice of 1 small lime
½ teaspoon chili powder
¼ teaspoon onion powder
¼ teaspoon garlic powder
6 tablespoons Dairy-Free Parmesan (page 36)
2 tablespoons chopped fresh cilantro

Preheat the grill to medium-high. Grill the corn for 8 to 12 minutes, turning occasionally, until the corn is cooked and charred on all sides. Transfer to a plate.

Meanwhile, in a small bowl, whisk together the mayonnaise, lime juice, chili powder, onion powder, and garlic powder.

Brush the sauce over each piece of grilled corn, then sprinkle all over with the dairy-free Parmesan. Garnish with the cilantro and serve.

*Make it easier:* No grill? No problem! Microwave the corn with the husks on: 4 minutes for a single ear; add 1 to 2 minutes for each additional ear, working in batches of 3 at a time. Proceed with the recipe as directed.

---

**Per Serving:** Calories: 257; Total fat: 18g; Carbohydrates: 22g; Cholesterol: 8mg; Fiber: 2.5g; Protein: 5g; Sugar: 7g

# CREAMY MASHED POTATOES

**Serves 4**
**Prep time: 10 minutes / Cook time: 15 minutes**

*Nut-Free, Vegetarian, Egg-Free Option, Gluten-Free Option, Soy-Free Option, Vegan Option*

These mashed potatoes are a great side for any occasion. Easy to whip up with just a few simple ingredients, they can also be customized to your liking–for example, by adding chives, chopped bacon, or fresh herbs. These are especially delicious topped with Mushroom and Sweet Onion Gravy (page 77).

2 pounds potatoes, peeled and cut into 2-inch chunks
3 tablespoons vegan butter
½ cup unsweetened oat milk (use certified gluten-free if needed) or other dairy-free milk
¼ cup mayonnaise
¼ teaspoon salt
¼ teaspoon freshly ground black pepper
¼ teaspoon garlic powder

1. Put the potatoes in a medium pot and add enough water to submerge the potatoes. Bring to a boil over high heat, then reduce the heat to medium and continue to boil for 10 to 12 minutes, or until the potatoes are tender. Drain the water, keeping the potatoes in the pot.

2. Add the butter, milk, mayonnaise, salt, pepper, and garlic powder and mash with a potato masher until the potatoes reach the desired texture.

*Substitution tip:* To make these egg-free, use a vegan mayonnaise in place of regular. To make soy-free, use a soy-free mayonnaise.

---

**Per Serving:** Calories: 358; Total fat: 20g; Carbohydrates: 41g; Cholesterol: 6mg; Fiber: 3.5g; Protein: 4g; Sugar: 3g

# HOMESTYLE DINNER ROLLS

**Makes 15 rolls**
**Prep time: 20 minutes, plus 35 minutes to rest / Cook time: 12 minutes**

*Egg-Free, Nut-Free, Soy-Free, Vegan*

In just a little more than an hour, you can have soft, fluffy homemade dinner rolls on your table. These rolls are the perfect accompaniment for just about any meal. Add a dollop of vegan butter or dip them in seasoned olive oil for a simple savory side. You can also use these rolls to make mini sliders, either with burgers, leftover holiday turkey, or Slow Cooker Pulled Pork (page 140).

1 tablespoon active dry yeast
1 cup warm water
¼ cup sugar
¼ cup unsweetened oat milk or other dairy-free milk
⅓ cup olive oil, plus more for greasing
½ teaspoon salt
3½ to 4 cups all-purpose flour, divided

In a large bowl, combine the yeast, warm water, and sugar. Let sit for 5 minutes, until it starts to become foamy.

Add the milk, oil, salt, and 2½ cups of flour. Mix using the dough hook attachment of a stand mixer or by hand until well combined. Continue to add the flour ½ cup at a time, until the dough is smooth and not sticky. Continue beating the dough on low speed for 2 to 3 minutes, or knead by hand for 2 to 3 minutes. Let the dough rest for 15 minutes.

Preheat the oven to 400°F. Grease a 9-by-13-inch baking dish with oil.

Divide the dough into 15 pieces, form them into balls, and place in the greased baking dish. Cover with a clean damp kitchen towel and let rest for 20 minutes, preferably over the center of the stovetop where ambient heat from the oven will help them rise.

Bake for 12 to 15 minutes, or until the tops are golden brown.

*Ingredient tip:* Even though active dry yeast is sold at room temperature at the grocery store, you should store it in the refrigerator or freezer after opening. If your yeast doesn't foam up in the first step, it's likely not good anymore, and your rolls won't rise properly.

---

**Per Serving (1 roll):** Calories: 172; Total fat: 5g; Carbohydrates: 28g; Cholesterol: 0mg; Fiber: 1g; Protein: 3g; Sugar: 3.5g

# CLASSIC HUMMUS

**Makes 1¼ cups**
**Prep time: 10 minutes**

*Egg-Free, Nut-Free, Soy-Free, Vegan, Gluten-Free Option*

It's incredibly simple to make your own hummus! The only unconventional ingredient you'll need is tahini, a paste made of ground sesame seeds. You can typically find this in the peanut butter section at your grocery store, or occasionally in the international section. If you can't find tahini, you can omit it and still make this–the hummus won't have the classic hint of sesame, but it still makes for a great dip.

1 (15.5-ounce) can chickpeas, rinsed and drained
1 garlic clove, peeled
¼ cup fresh lemon juice
3 tablespoons tahini
3 tablespoons extra-virgin olive oil
½ teaspoon salt
¼ teaspoon ground cumin
Vegetables or pita bread (gluten-free brand if needed), for serving

1. In a food processor, combine the chickpeas, garlic, lemon juice, tahini, oil, salt, and cumin and process for 60 to 90 seconds, or until the hummus is smooth.
2. Serve with chopped vegetables or warm pita bread. Store leftover hummus in the refrigerator for up to 4 days.

*Mix it up:* Hummus can be used for more than just dip. Try mixing it into grain bowls to add creaminess and flavor, like in the Greek Rice and Veggie Bowls (page 105). You can also toss cooked vegetables in hummus, or use it as a "sauce" for pizza.

---

**Per Serving (2 tablespoons, without vegetables or bread):** Calories: 101; Total fat: 7g; Carbohydrates: 8g; Cholesterol: 0mg; Fiber: 2g; Protein: 3g; Sugar: 1g

# FRENCH ONION DIP

**Makes about 1½ cups**
**Prep time: 10 minutes, plus 2 hours to thicken**

Score a touchdown on game day by mixing up this dip. With just three simple ingredients, you won't believe how much this resembles traditional French onion dip. Though it might be tempting to skip the cheesecloth step in the recipe, letting the mixture sit for a few hours ensures that the excess liquid drains out of the yogurt, creating the thick consistency of sour cream.

1½ cups almond milk yogurt
2½ tablespoons fresh lemon juice
1 (1-ounce) packet onion soup mix (check to ensure dairy-free)
Potato chips or sliced vegetables, for serving

Cover a medium bowl securely with cheesecloth. In another medium bowl, stir together the yogurt and lemon juice. Pour this mixture on top of the cheesecloth. Let sit in the refrigerator for at least 2 hours, or overnight, to thicken.

Once thickened, scoop what's left on the cheesecloth into another bowl, discarding any drained liquid. Stir in the onion soup mix until well combined.

Serve with chips or vegetables for dipping. Store any leftover dip covered in the refrigerator for up to 4 days. Stir well before using again.

*Mix it up:* If you have other dip recipes that use sour cream as a base, you can use this same method to make those. Also, try swapping out the onion soup mix and instead mixing in caramelized onions, bacon, chives, salt, pepper, and garlic powder.

---

**Per Serving (¼ cup, without dippers):** Calories: 51; Total fat: 2.5g; Carbohydrates: 7g; Cholesterol: 0mg; Fiber: 1.5g; Protein: 1g; Sugar: 3g

# SAVORY HOMEMADE CRACKERS

**Makes about 100 small crackers**
**Prep time: 20 minutes / Cook time: 15 minutes**

*Egg-Free, Nut-Free, Soy-Free, Vegan*

Many store-bought crackers are dairy-free, but it's always nice to know how to make your own. These are a bit of a cross between a classic buttery cracker and a cheese cracker—the nutritional yeast adds a subtle cheesiness, and the other seasonings enhance the flavor. I love to add a few shakes of cayenne for a hint of spice, but it's up to you.

- 1 cup all-purpose flour, plus more for sprinkling
- 2 tablespoons nutritional yeast
- ½ teaspoon salt
- ½ teaspoon garlic powder
- ½ teaspoon paprika
- ⅛ teaspoon cayenne pepper (optional)
- 4 tablespoons vegan butter, at room temperature
- 2 teaspoons fresh lemon juice
- 3 to 6 tablespoons cold water

1. Preheat the oven to 350°F.
2. In a large bowl, combine the flour, nutritional yeast, salt, garlic powder, paprika, and cayenne (if using). Stir well, then mix in the butter and lemon juice. The dough will be crumbly and dry. Mix in the water, 1 tablespoon at a time, until the mixture forms a cohesive dough.
3. Use your hands to form the dough into a disk, then place it on a lightly floured piece of parchment paper. Sprinkle flour over the top, then roll the dough out as thin as you can, 1⁄16 to ⅛ inch thick. Use a knife or a pizza cutter to gently cut the dough into small squares.
4. Transfer the parchment paper with the cracker squares onto the baking sheet. Bake for 15 to 20 minutes, or until golden brown and crisp. Let cool before transferring to an airtight container. Store at room temperature for up to 1 week.

*Cooking tip:* The thinner you roll your dough, the quicker the crackers will cook and the crispier they will be. Keep an eye on them closely while cooking, as they can progress from perfectly cooked to burnt in just a few minutes!

**Per Serving (10 crackers):** Calories: 88; Total fat: 5g; Carbohydrates: 10g; Cholesterol: 0mg; Fiber: 1g; Protein: 2g; Sugar: 0g

# CHILI-LIME POPCORN

**Makes about 14 cups**
**Prep time: 5 minutes / Cook time: 10 minutes**

*Egg-Free, Gluten-Free, Nut-Free, Soy-Free, Vegan*

If you've got kids, they'll love seeing this "old-fashioned" way of making popcorn on the stovetop. Fresh popped popcorn is incredibly easy to make; it takes just a few minutes for the oil to heat up and then a few more to pop the kernels. You can just toss the popcorn with salt afterward; however, the chili-lime seasoning in this recipe adds a fun zesty pop (pun intended) of flavor.

4 tablespoons olive oil or coconut oil, divided
½ cup popcorn kernels
Grated zest and juice of 1 lime
1 teaspoon chili powder
1 teaspoon salt

Pour 2 tablespoons of oil into a large pot and add 2 or 3 individual popcorn kernels. Set the pot over medium heat, partially cover, and wait for the kernels to pop.

When they pop, pour in the remainder of the popcorn, giving the pot a little shake to ensure all the popcorn is evenly coated. Partially cover the pot again. The popcorn will start popping fairly quickly. Continue cooking until the sound slows to a few seconds between pops. Pour the popcorn into a large bowl.

In the same pot, heat the remaining 2 tablespoons of oil over medium heat. Stir in the lime zest, lime juice, chili powder, and salt. Cook for about 30 seconds, then pour over the popcorn and toss well to combine.

Store any leftover popcorn in an airtight bag at room temperature. For best quality, enjoy within 5 days.

*Mix it up:* Here are some other delicious seasoning ideas that can be used with the basic stovetop popcorn method: 1) vegan butter and salt; 2) olive oil, nutritional yeast, garlic powder, and salt; 3) vegan butter, brown sugar, cinnamon, and salt; or 4) chopped bacon and maple syrup.

---

**Per Serving (1 cup):** Calories: 65; Total fat: 4g; Carbohydrates: 6g; Cholesterol: 0mg; Fiber: 1g; Protein: 1g; Sugar: 0g

# ENERGY BITES WITH CRANBERRY, COCONUT, AND CHIA SEEDS

**Makes 15 energy bites**
**Prep time: 10 minutes**

*Egg-Free, Gluten-Free Option, Soy-Free, Vegetarian*

Energy bites are a cross between an energy snack and a dessert. Lightly sweetened with honey, they also contain nutritious ingredients. The oats provide energy-fueling carbs and digestive-friendly fiber, and the walnuts and chia seeds supply healthy fats for cardiovascular health. Prep these ahead of time and grab-and-go as needed throughout the week, or pack them for a snack during a weekend hike.

¾ cup rolled oats (certified gluten-free if needed)
¾ cup pitted dates
½ cup walnuts
½ cup dried cranberries
¼ cup unsweetened shredded coconut
¼ cup honey
2 tablespoons chia seeds

In a food processor, combine all the ingredients and process for 30 to 60 seconds, until the mixture is well combined and starts to clump together. Roll into 15 balls (about 1 inch in diameter). Store in the refrigerator for up to 5 days.

*Mix it up:* Energy bites can be customized to include the flavors you enjoy and ingredients you have on hand. Start with a base of oats, dates or golden raisins, and nuts or nut butter, then add onto that. Try this apple peanut butter combination: 1 cup rolled oats, ½ cup peanut butter, ½ cup dates, 1 chopped apple, 1 tablespoon chia seeds, and 1 teaspoon cinnamon. For a lemon energy bite, try ½ cup rolled oats, ½ cup roasted cashews, ⅓ cup golden raisins, zest and juice of 1 lemon, ¼ cup shredded coconut, and 1 tablespoon chia seeds.

---

**Per Serving (1 bite):** Calories: 100; Total fat: 4g; Carbohydrates: 17g; Cholesterol: 0mg; Fiber: 2g; Protein: 2g; Sugar: 12g

# FROZEN BANANA BITES

**Makes about 30 bites**
**Prep time: 20 minutes, plus 2 to 3 hours to freeze**

*Egg-Free, Gluten-Free, Soy-Free, Vegan*

The pairing of fruit and peanut butter delivers a great balance of protein, carbs, and healthy fats to keep you satisfied and energized. Jazz up this classic snack-time combo by making these frozen banana bites. Freezing the banana peanut butter "sandwich" provides a different textural experience, reminiscent of a frozen dessert bar. Dip them in dark chocolate for a truly indulgent sweet treat.

- 3 bananas, cut into ¼-inch-thick slices
- ⅓ cup peanut butter
- 1 cup dairy-free dark chocolate chips (optional)

1. Line a baking sheet with parchment paper. Place half the banana slices on the parchment paper and spread peanut butter on top of each banana slice. Place the remaining banana slices on top, creating mini "sandwiches."
2. Put the baking sheet in the freezer for 1 to 2 hours, or until the bites are frozen. If you plan to eat as is, remove from the baking sheet and place in a zip-top bag to store in the freezer.
3. If covering in chocolate, melt the chocolate chips in the microwave in 20-second increments, stirring after each, until the chocolate has just melted. Dip each banana bite in chocolate and place back on the parchment paper. Return the baking sheet to the freezer for 1 hour, then move the bites into a freezer-safe bag.

*Mix it up:* Instead of peanut butter and chocolate, you can also make frozen banana bites with dairy-free yogurt. Slice the bananas a bit thicker, ½- to 1-inch pieces, and dip in your favorite dairy-free yogurt. Freeze for 2 hours. I love these in a vanilla coconut milk yogurt.

---

**Per Serving (3 bites):** Calories: 82; Total fat: 4.5g; Carbohydrates: 10g; Cholesterol: 0mg; Fiber: 1.5g; Protein: 2g; Sugar: 5g

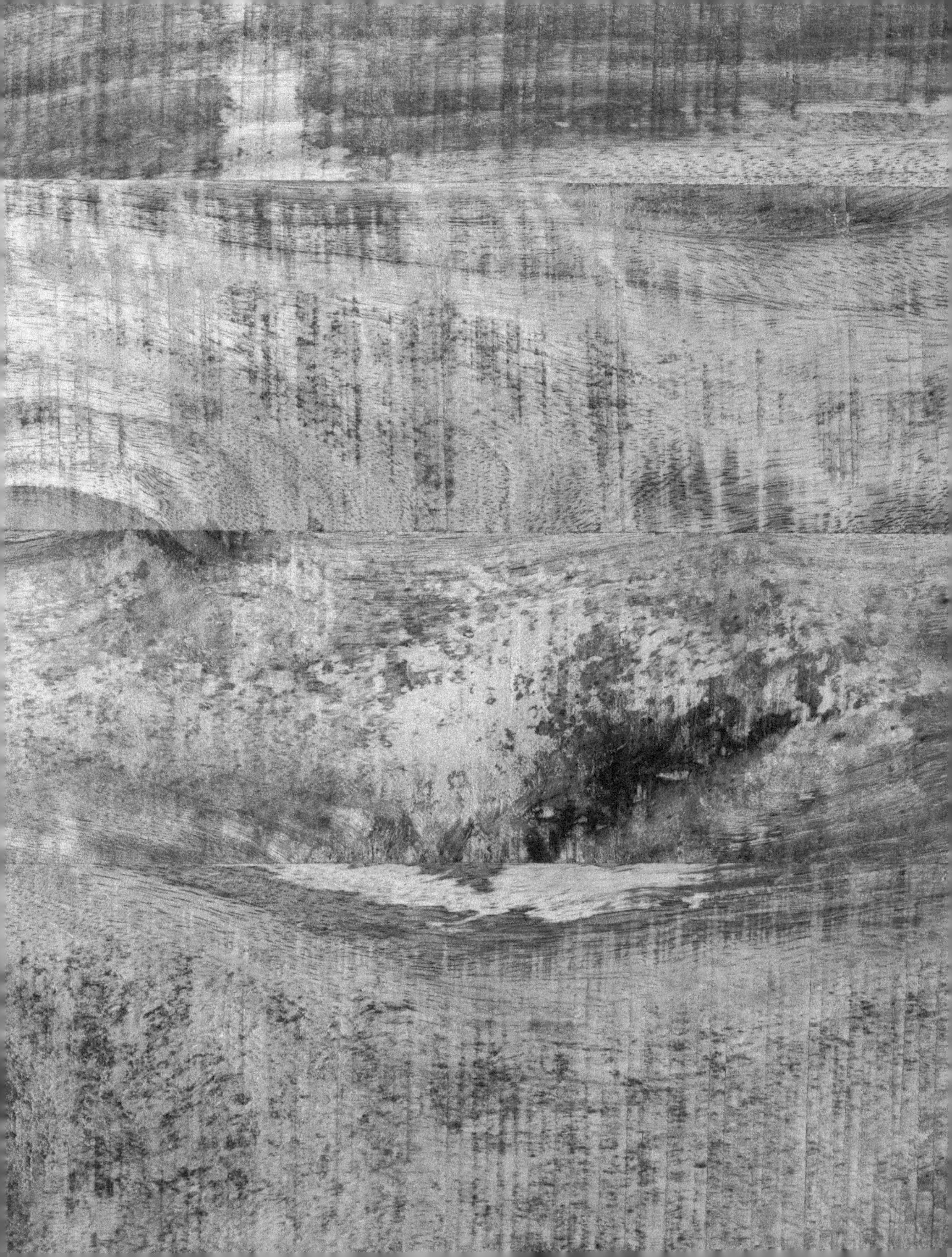

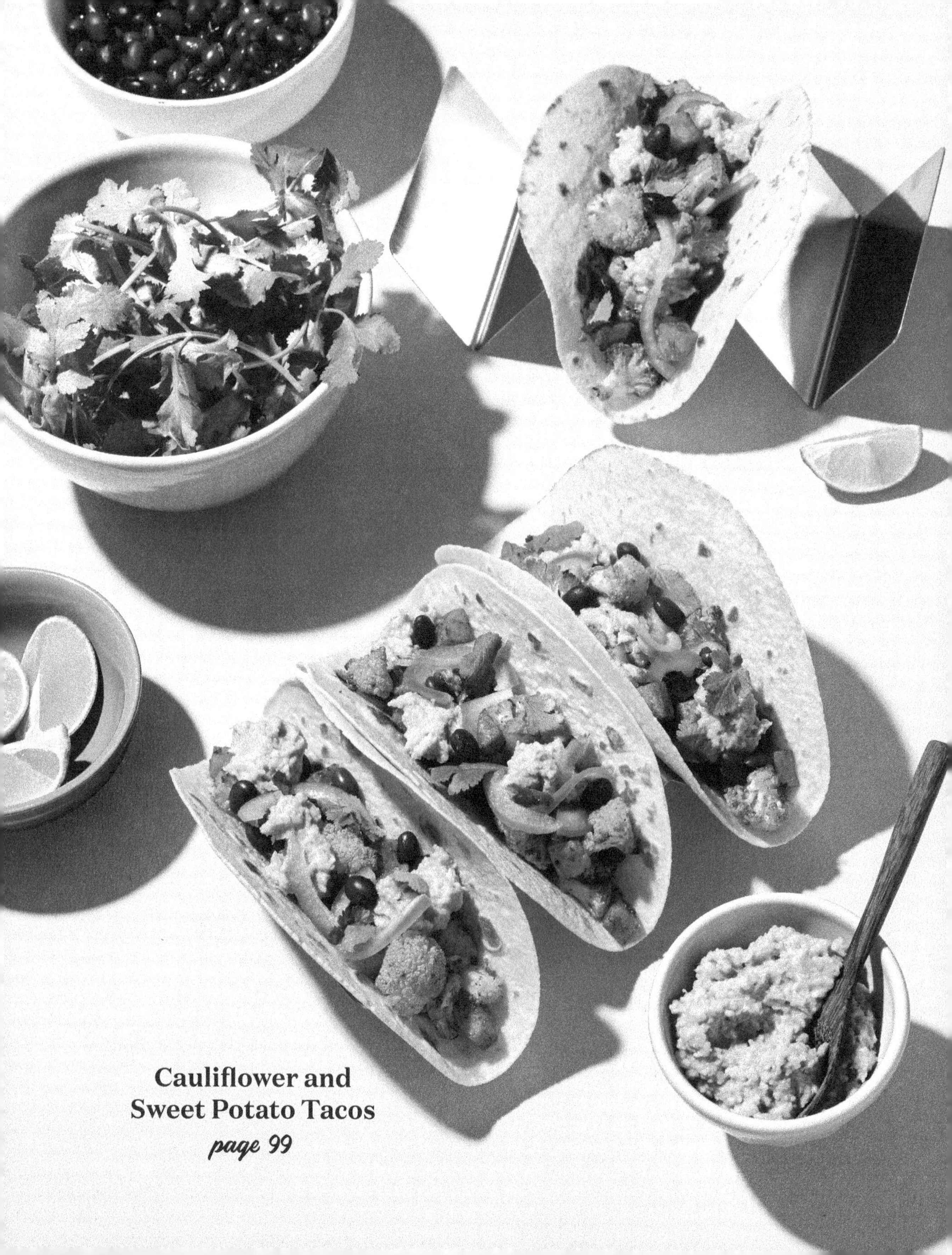

**Cauliflower and Sweet Potato Tacos**

*page 99*

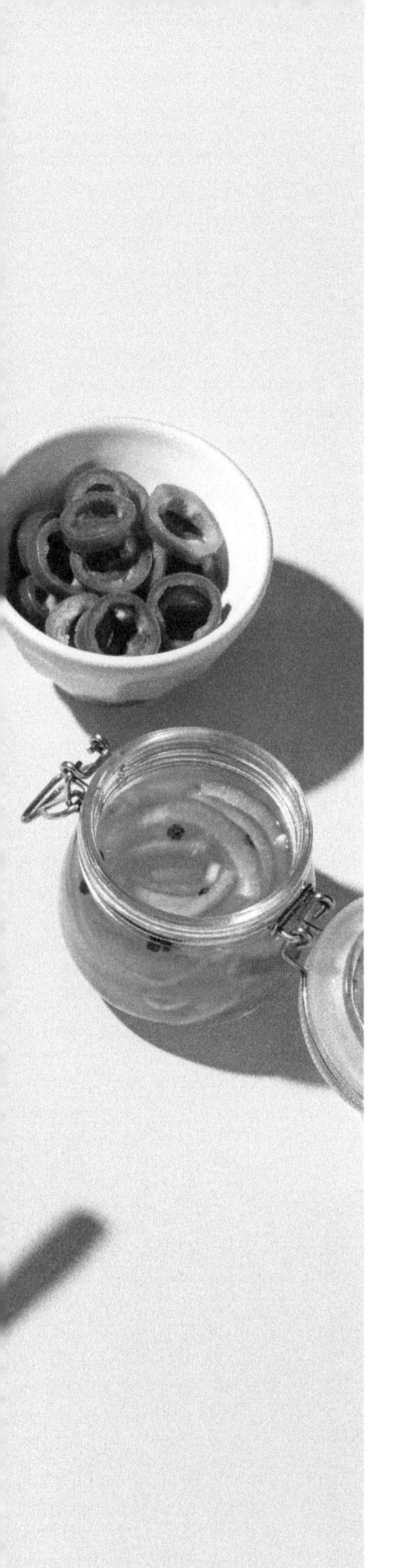

Seven

# Vegetarian and Vegan Dishes

# PESTO ZOODLES

**Serves 4**

**Prep time: 15 minutes / Cook time: 5 minutes**

*Egg-Free, Gluten-Free, Soy-Free, Vegan, Nut-Free Option (see tip)*

Many of my friends have been gifted with a knack for gardening, growing beautiful heirloom vegetables and fresh herbs. Unfortunately, I was not gifted with such a green thumb, but basil is one plant that I can pretty much always grow successfully. Fresh basil tastes fantastic in homemade pesto, which can easily be made dairy-free by omitting Parmesan cheese from traditional recipes. Toss the pesto together with zucchini noodles and serve alongside crusty bread for a light summer meal.

**For the pesto**

2 cups fresh basil leaves
2 garlic cloves, peeled
¼ cup walnuts
¼ cup olive oil
1 tablespoon nutritional yeast
¼ teaspoon salt

**For the zoodles**

1 tablespoon olive oil
5 or 6 medium zucchini, peeled and spiralized

1. **To make the pesto:** In the bowl of a small food processor, combine the basil, garlic, walnuts, oil, nutritional yeast, and salt. Process for 30 to 40 seconds, until well blended.

2. **To make the zoodles:** In a large skillet, heat the oil over medium heat. Add the zucchini noodles and cook for 3 to 4 minutes, stirring often, until the zucchini is crisp-tender.

   Remove from the heat and drain any liquid in the pan. Add the pesto and toss to coat. Serve immediately.

*Ingredient tip:* If you don't own a spiralizer, run a peeler over your zucchini repeatedly, forming pappardelle-style noodles. Also, these zucchini noodles do not store or reheat well, so only use as much zucchini as you need for the meal. Save any extra pesto to use another night for freshly cooked zoodles, pasta, pizza, or sandwiches.

*Protein swap:* Swap the walnuts for other nuts, like cashews or almonds. You can also use pumpkin seeds to make this a nut-free dish.

---

**Per Serving:** Calories 242; Total fat: 22g; Carbohydrates: 10g; Cholesterol: 0mg; Fiber: 3g; Protein: 5g; Sugar: 6g

# PLANTAIN FRITTATA

**Serves 6**
**Prep time: 15 minutes / Cook time: 35 minutes**

*Gluten-Free, Soy-Free, Vegetarian*

Frittatas aren't just for breakfast—they make a lovely dinner, especially served alongside a big salad. Plantains aren't typically used in frittatas here in the United States; it's more common to see this pairing in other countries. Plantains bear a resemblance to bananas and come from the same plant family. However, they are much starchier than bananas and are cooked before eating. Here, we'll fry the plantains first, then layer them on top of the egg mixture prior to baking.

3 tablespoons canola oil
1 yellow plantain, peeled and cut into ¼-inch slices
⅛ teaspoon salt, plus ¼ teaspoon, divided
½ yellow onion, chopped
½ large bell pepper (any color), chopped
1 cup chopped tomatoes
8 large eggs
¼ cup unsweetened almond milk or other dairy-free milk

1. Preheat the oven to 375°F.
2. In a cast iron or other ovenproof skillet, heat the oil over medium heat. Add the plantain in a single layer, working in batches if necessary, panfrying for 2 to 3 minutes per side. Remove with a slotted spoon and set aside on paper towels to drain, sprinkling with ⅛ teaspoon of salt.
3. Add the onion and bell pepper to the oil remaining in the skillet and cook over medium heat, stirring occasionally, for about 5 minutes, or until tender. Stir in the tomatoes and remove from the heat.
4. In a large bowl, whisk together the eggs, almond milk, and remaining ¼ teaspoon of salt. Pour the egg mixture into the skillet with the onion and pepper. Arrange the plantain in a single layer on top.
5. Transfer to the oven and bake for 15 to 20 minutes, or until the eggs are set and a knife pulls out clean from the center.

Cut into wedges to serve. Store leftovers in the refrigerator for up to 4 days. Reheat in the microwave.

*Substitution tip:* If you don't have an ovenproof skillet, use a regular skillet to prepare the vegetables. Transfer the vegetables and whisked eggs to a baking dish, top with the plantain, and bake.

---

**Per Serving:** Calories: 207; Total fat: 14g; Carbohydrates: 13g; Cholesterol: 248mg; Fiber: 1.5g; Protein: 9g; Sugar: 6g

# CORN AND SWEET POTATO FRITTERS

**Makes 10 fritters**
**Prep time: 15 minutes / Cook time: 20 minutes**

*Nut-Free, Vegetarian*

These corn and sweet potato fritters are a little unconventional, but they taste great—especially when topped with garlic aioli. A true aioli is made with just olive oil and garlic, but we're cheating to make it easier with a mayonnaise-based version. Don't be intimidated by the longer ingredient list in this recipe. It's mostly pantry staples, and prep just involves tossing your ingredients in a bowl and shaping the fritters. Easy-peasy!

**For the aioli**
½ cup mayonnaise
2 teaspoons minced garlic
1 teaspoon Dijon mustard
1 teaspoon apple cider vinegar
½ teaspoon salt
⅛ teaspoon freshly ground black pepper

**For the fritters**
2 medium sweet potatoes
1 cup canned corn kernels, drained (or kernels from 2 ears fresh corn)
2 scallions, chopped
¼ cup chopped fresh cilantro
½ cup yellow cornmeal
¼ cup all-purpose flour
¼ cup unsweetened oat milk
1½ teaspoons ground cumin
½ teaspoon salt
⅛ teaspoon cayenne pepper
¼ cup canola oil, plus up to 3 tablespoons more if needed

1. **To make the aioli:** In a small bowl, combine the mayonnaise, garlic, mustard, vinegar, salt, and pepper. Stir until well combined and set aside.
2. **To make the fritters:** Poke a few holes in the sweet potatoes with a fork and place them in a bowl. Cover with a wet paper towel and microwave for 6 to 10 minutes, or until tender. Remove and let cool.
3. Meanwhile, in a large bowl, combine the corn, scallions, cilantro, cornmeal, flour, milk, cumin, salt, and cayenne.
4. When the sweet potatoes are cool, peel them and add the flesh to the bowl. Mix until well combined, using the back of a fork to mash the potatoes.
5. In a large skillet, heat the oil over medium heat. Shape the fritter mixture into 10 patties. Working in two batches so as not to overcrowd the pan, cook the fritters for about 2 minutes per side, or until golden brown on each side. Remove and place on paper towels to drain. If needed, add extra oil to the pan for the second batch.

Serve the fritters immediately, topped with the aioli. Store leftover fritters and aioli separately in the refrigerator for up to 4 days. Reheat the fritters in a 350°F oven for 10 minutes, until crisp.

*Make it easier:* Look for a premade garlic aioli at the grocery store.

---

**Per Serving (1 fritter):** Calories: 221; Total fat: 17g; Carbohydrates: 17g; Cholesterol: 5mg; Fiber: 1.5g; Protein: 2g; Sugar: 2.5g

# CAULIFLOWER AND SWEET POTATO TACOS

**Makes 10 tacos**
**Prep time: 20 minutes / Cook time: 30 minutes**

*Egg-Free, Nut-Free, Soy-Free, Vegan*

Impress your guests with these restaurant-quality vegan tacos. Roasting the sweet potatoes and cauliflower caramelizes their natural sugars, creating a depth of flavor that tastes wonderful in a warm, charred corn tortilla. These tacos are topped with fresh guacamole and pickled red onions, which add richness and acidity to make for a well-rounded dish. You can easily scale up and double this recipe if you're making it for a crowd.

1 head cauliflower, cut into bite-size florets
2 medium sweet potatoes, peeled and cut into bite-size pieces
2 tablespoons olive oil
½ teaspoon salt
½ teaspoon ground cumin
½ teaspoon chili powder
¼ teaspoon freshly ground black pepper
2 avocados, halved and pitted
Juice of 1 lime
10 corn tortillas
1 cup canned black beans, rinsed and drained
½ cup Quick-Pickled Red Onions (page 78)
¼ cup chopped fresh cilantro

1. Preheat the oven to 425°F.
2. Arrange the cauliflower and sweet potatoes on a sheet pan. Drizzle with the oil and sprinkle with the salt, cumin, chili powder, and pepper, then rub the vegetables around the pan to fully coat them. Bake for 25 to 30 minutes, or until the sweet potatoes are tender and the cauliflower is caramelized on the edges.
3. Meanwhile, scoop the avocados into a bowl and mash with the lime juice to make a simple guacamole.
4. Warm the corn tortillas by placing them, one at a time, over the direct flame of a gas stove or in a hot skillet. When they get a little charred on the bottom (15 to 60 seconds, depending on which method you're using), flip them with tongs to warm the other side. Place them on a plate and cover with a slightly damp paper towel until you're ready to use them.

Load up each tortilla with the cooked cauliflower and potatoes, guacamole, black beans, pickled red onions, and cilantro. Serve immediately.

*Ingredient tip:* Avocados brown quickly, so if dinner gets delayed, cover the guacamole with plastic wrap, pressing down to adhere the plastic to the surface of the guac.

*Mix it up:* Experiment with different vegetable and bean combinations for an endless variety of vegan tacos. For example, try sautéed mushrooms and jalapeños with black beans, or roasted zucchini and bell peppers with pinto beans.

---

**Per Serving (2 tacos):** Calories: 404; Total fat: 16g; Carbohydrates: 59g; Cholesterol: 0mg; Fiber: 14g; Protein: 11g; Sugar: 8.5g

# MEXICAN-INSPIRED STUFFED SWEET POTATOES

**Serves 4**
**Prep time: 15 minutes / Cook time: 40 minutes**

*Egg-Free, Vegan*

Stuffed sweet potatoes can accommodate an endless variety of toppings, and one of our family favorites has always been a Mexican-style spin. I traditionally make this dish with seasoned ground beef, but then I discovered a fun way to make this vegan—using pecan "taco meat"! When processed in a food processor with seasonings, pecans take on a texture and flavor reminiscent of traditional taco meat. Load this great mixture onto a sweet potato with beans, corn, and tomatoes, and you've got a unique meatless meal that really satisfies.

**For the sweet potatoes**
4 large sweet potatoes, each poked with a fork a few times
1 tablespoon olive oil

**For the pecan "taco meat"**
1 cup pecans or walnuts
1 tablespoon soy sauce
½ teaspoon ground cumin
½ teaspoon chili powder
½ teaspoon paprika
¼ teaspoon garlic powder

**For the stuffing**
½ cup canned black beans, rinsed and drained
½ cup canned corn kernels, rinsed and drained
½ cup cherry tomatoes, halved
Guacamole (optional)

1. **To make the sweet potatoes:** Preheat the oven to 400°F.
2. Place the sweet potatoes on a baking sheet and drizzle with the oil; then roll them around the pan to evenly coat. Bake for 40 to 50 minutes, or until tender.
3. **Meanwhile, to make the pecan "taco meat":** In a food processor, combine the pecans, soy sauce, cumin, chili powder, paprika, and garlic powder. Pulse several times until the texture resembles crumbled ground meat.
4. **To stuff the sweet potatoes:** Slit the sweet potatoes open lengthwise and top with the pecan taco mixture, beans, corn, and tomatoes. Top with guacamole (if using). Store leftovers in the refrigerator for up to 4 days. Reheat in the microwave.

*Make it easier:* Instead of baking the sweet potatoes, cook them in the microwave. Poke them with a fork a few times, then place 2 at a time in a microwave-safe bowl and cover with a damp paper towel. Cook for 6 to 8 minutes, or until tender. Repeat for the remaining 2 potatoes. Proceed with the recipe as directed.

---

**Per Serving:** Calories: 360; Total fat: 22g; Carbohydrates: 38g; Cholesterol: 0mg; Fiber: 9g; Protein: 7g; Sugar: 8g

# PORTOBELLO SHEET PAN FAJITAS

**Makes 8 fajitas**
**Prep time: 15 minutes / Cook time: 25 minutes**

These vegetarian fajitas employ portobello mushrooms for the base of the dish, a vegetable with an almost meaty texture and earthy, umami flavor. The mushrooms, peppers, and onion make for a simple-yet-hearty filling for fajitas. I like to make a quick homemade guacamole with avocado and lime to add to these, but you can also use store-bought guac to make this meal even easier.

4 large portobello caps (about 12 ounces), gills scraped out, cut into ½-inch-thick slices
3 medium bell peppers (any color), sliced
1 yellow onion, sliced
2 tablespoons olive oil
½ teaspoon salt
½ teaspoon chili powder
½ teaspoon ground cumin
2 avocados, halved and pitted
Juice of 2 limes
8 (6-inch) flour tortillas

Preheat the oven to 400°F.

Arrange the mushrooms, bell peppers, and onion on a sheet pan. (Use two sheet pans if it doesn't all fit on one.) Drizzle with the oil and sprinkle with the salt, chili powder, and cumin. Gently toss the vegetables to evenly coat. Bake for 24 to 28 minutes, or until the vegetables are tender.

Meanwhile, scoop the avocados into a bowl and mash with the lime juice to make a quick guacamole.

Divide the vegetables among the tortillas and top with guacamole. Serve immediately.

*Substitution tip:* Make this recipe gluten-free by purchasing gluten-free tortillas.

---

**Per Serving (2 fajitas):** Calories: 421; Total fat: 23g; Carbohydrates: 48g; Cholesterol: 0mg; Fiber: 9.5g; Protein: 10g; Sugar: 7.5g

# MUSHROOM RAMEN

**Serves 4**
**Prep time: 10 minutes / Cook time: 35 minutes**

*Nut-Free, Vegetarian, Gluten-Free Option (see tip), Soy-Free Option*

This mushroom ramen offers a step up from plain instant noodles by adding fresh vegetables and a perfect soft-boiled egg. Double-check the ramen that you're purchasing. Many varieties contain dairy in the seasoning packets, which you'll discard for this recipe. However, it's wise to also double-check that the noodles are dairy-free. If you have a serious dairy allergy, look for brands that do not risk cross-contamination with the seasoning packets.

4 large eggs
1 tablespoon toasted sesame oil or olive oil
2 garlic cloves, minced
½ tablespoon minced fresh ginger
1 (8-ounce) package sliced baby bella (cremini) mushrooms
½ cup sliced shiitake mushrooms
1 tablespoon soy sauce
4 cups vegetable broth
3 cups packed baby spinach
2 (3-ounce) packages ramen noodles, seasoning packets discarded
3 scallions, chopped

1. Bring a small pot of water to a boil. Slowly lower the eggs into the pot and boil for 7 minutes. Drain and run the eggs under cool tap water, then set aside.

2. Meanwhile, in a soup pot, heat the sesame oil over medium heat. Add the garlic and ginger and cook, stirring frequently, for 2 to 3 minutes. Add both mushrooms and cook, stirring occasionally, for another 6 to 8 minutes, until the mushrooms have started to soften.

3. Add the soy sauce and broth and simmer for 10 minutes. Stir in the spinach and ramen and cook for 3 to 4 minutes, or until the spinach is wilted and the ramen is cooked through.

4. Divide the soup evenly among four bowls, topping with the scallions. Peel and slice the soft-boiled eggs, add one to each bowl, and enjoy.

*Substitution tip:* To make this soy-free and gluten-free, switch out the soy sauce for coconut aminos, and purchase soy- and gluten-free ramen noodles (available at some grocery stores and online).

---

**Per Serving:** Calories: 245; Total fat: 12g; Carbohydrates: 21g; Cholesterol: 186mg; Fiber: 3g; Protein: 12g; Sugar: 4g

# RICE NOODLE STIR-FRY

**Serves 4**
**Prep time: 15 minutes / Cook time: 15 minutes**

*Egg-Free, Vegan, Gluten-Free Option, Soy-Free Option (see tip)*

Stir-fry recipes are great "clean out the fridge" meals. Just combine any vegetables you want to use up, along with a noodle or rice of your choice, and toss with a delicious sauce. In this recipe, I went with peppers, mushrooms, carrots, and cabbage, but use what you've got on hand. If you decide to make this exactly as directed, save yourself time by purchasing preshredded cabbage (sometimes labeled "coleslaw mix") and pregrated carrots at the grocery store.

**For the sauce**
¼ cup soy sauce
¼ cup vegetable broth
2 tablespoons brown sugar
1 tablespoon rice vinegar
1 tablespoon toasted sesame oil
1 teaspoon cornstarch

**For the stir-fry**
7 ounces dried rice noodles
1 tablespoon olive oil
1 bell pepper (any color), chopped
1½ cups sliced baby bella (cremini) mushrooms
½ cup grated carrots
2 cups shredded cabbage

**For garnishes (optional)**
Roasted cashews
Chopped cilantro

**To make the sauce:** In a medium bowl, whisk together the soy sauce, broth, brown sugar, vinegar, sesame oil, and cornstarch. Set aside.

**To make the stir-fry:** Cook the rice noodles according to package directions. Drain and set aside.

Meanwhile, in a large skillet, heat the olive oil over medium heat. Add the bell pepper and mushrooms and cook, stirring occasionally, for 4 minutes. Add the carrots and cook, stirring occasionally, for another 2 minutes. Add the cabbage and cook, stirring occasionally, for 2 more minutes.

Add the noodles to the skillet and pour the sauce over the top. Toss everything together to combine and let cook for 2 to 3 minutes to thicken the sauce up a bit.

Serve immediately. If desired, top with cashews and cilantro. Store leftovers in the refrigerator for up to 4 days.

*Substitution tip:* Make this dish gluten-free by switching out the soy sauce for tamari, and checking to ensure the rice noodles are gluten-free (occasionally they contain wheat). To make this dish soy-free, use coconut aminos rather than soy sauce and reduce the brown sugar to 1 tablespoon.

---

**Per Serving:** Calories: 302; Total fat: 8g; Carbohydrates: 54g; Cholesterol: 0mg; Fiber: 3g; Protein: 5g; Sugar: 11g

# GREEK RICE AND VEGGIE BOWLS

**Serves 4**
**Prep time: 15 minutes / Cook time: 20 to 40 minutes**

*Egg-Free, Gluten-Free, Nut-Free, Soy-Free, Vegetarian*

Although rice and veggies may seem a little boring at first glance, don't be fooled–these Greek bowls are anything but mundane! Tossing the ingredients with hummus adds flavor and creaminess to this dish, and the roasted red peppers and pickled red onions deliver unexpected pops of flavor with every bite. This is a great meal prep recipe that can be served warm or cold.

- 1 cup long-grain white or brown rice
- 1 pint cherry tomatoes, halved
- 1 cucumber, peeled and chopped
- 1 cup packed baby spinach
- ¾ cup Classic Hummus (page 85)
- ⅔ cup chopped jarred roasted red peppers
- ⅔ cup Quick-Pickled Red Onions (page 78)

1. Cook the rice according to package directions.
2. In a large bowl, combine the warm cooked rice, tomatoes, cucumber, spinach, hummus, roasted peppers, and pickled onions. Mix well and serve immediately. Store leftovers in the refrigerator for up to 4 days.

*Protein swap:* This meal also tastes great with cooked chicken or turkey breast. You can also swap out the rice for quinoa.

---

**Per Serving:** Calories: 370; Total fat: 11g; Carbohydrates: 59g; Cholesterol: 0mg; Fiber: 5.5g; Protein: 9g; Sugar: 9.5g

# ARUGULA LEMON PASTA

**Serves 4**
**Prep time: 10 minutes / Cook time: 15 minutes**

*Egg-Free, Soy-Free, Vegan, Gluten-Free Option*

Hands-down, a big bowl of spaghetti and meatballs is my family's favorite pasta dish, but for me, this arugula lemon pasta ranks high on my list of preferred pastas. It's very simple to make, especially if you already have leftover Italian-Style Cashew Ricotta from another recipe. The peppery arugula pairs nicely with the citrusy lemon, and it all comes together with the creamy ricotta sauce.

8 ounces farfalle or rotini pasta (use gluten-free if needed)
¾ cup Italian-Style Cashew Ricotta (page 37)
¾ cup unsweetened almond milk or other dairy-free milk
½ teaspoon salt
2 cups packed baby arugula
Grated zest and juice of 1 lemon
Dairy-Free Parmesan (optional, page 36)

Cook the pasta in a large pot according to package directions. Drain.

In the same pot, heat the ricotta, milk, and salt, whisking until well combined. Stir in the arugula, lemon zest, lemon juice, and drained pasta. Cook for 1 to 2 minutes, constantly tossing the ingredients until everything is well mixed.

Serve immediately. Top with dairy-free Parmesan (if using). Store leftovers covered in the refrigerator for up to 4 days.

*Substitution tip:* Swap in different greens of your choice. Instead of arugula, try baby spinach or baby kale.

---

**Per Serving:** Calories: 393; Total fat: 14g; Carbohydrates: 53g; Cholesterol: 0mg; Fiber: 4g; Protein: 14g; Sugar: 3g

# MAC AND CHEESE

**Serves 4**

**Prep time: 10 minutes / Cook time: 15 minutes**

*Egg-Free, Vegan, Nut-Free Option, Soy-Free Option*

Macaroni and cheese is one of the more difficult meals to re-create on a dairy-free diet. Dairy-free cheeses taste and melt differently than their dairy-based counterparts, and the quality varies considerably across different brands. However, when you find a high-quality dairy-free cheddar cheese, you'll be happy to have this recipe. I personally make this with Violife dairy-free shredded cheddar, and it's pretty much the closest thing you can get to "real" mac and cheese: creamy, gooey, and rich in flavor. Definitely worth the effort.

8 ounces elbow macaroni
1½ tablespoons olive oil
½ yellow onion, chopped
1 teaspoon minced garlic
2 tablespoons all-purpose flour
¾ cup unsweetened oat milk or other dairy-free milk
¾ cup vegetable broth or chicken broth
1 (8-ounce) package shredded dairy-free cheddar cheese (nut-free or soy-free if needed)

1. Cook the pasta according to package directions. Drain and set aside.
2. Meanwhile, in a large sauté pan or skillet, heat the oil over medium heat. Add the onion and cook, stirring occasionally, for 4 to 5 minutes, or until it starts to get tender. Add the garlic and cook, stirring, for another minute.
3. Stir in the flour, letting it coat the onion and garlic, and cook for 30 seconds. Slowly whisk in the milk and broth, adding a little at a time, mixing thoroughly with the flour to let it thicken up.
4. Add the cheddar, stirring often. Continue cooking for 2 to 3 minutes, or until the cheese is fully melted and incorporated into the sauce. Stir in the drained macaroni and toss everything together until well combined. Serve immediately.

*Ingredient tip:* Not all dairy-free cheeses will taste the same raw as they do when mixed into a recipe. Some brands taste better when mixed with other flavors in a finished dish. Experiment until you find what works for you.

---

**Per Serving:** Calories: 405; Total fat: 17g; Carbohydrates: 54g; Cholesterol: 0mg; Fiber: 5g; Protein: 10g; Sugar: 4g

# STUFFED SHELLS

**Serves 5**

**Prep time: 10 minutes / Cook time: 35 minutes**

Kid-friendly Italian favorites were always in our meal rotation when I was growing up. From lasagna to spaghetti and meatballs to stuffed shells, my siblings and I loved 'em all. Thankfully, the dairy-free versions of these classic dishes are super satisfying, and these stuffed shells are proof of that. Filled with creamy Italian-Style Cashew Ricotta and spinach, no one will even guess that these don't contain cheese. If you find a dairy-free mozzarella cheese that you like, you can add that as a topping before baking, but I find they're great as is.

6 ounces jumbo pasta shells (use gluten-free if needed)
1 (10-ounce) package frozen chopped spinach, thawed
Italian-Style Cashew Ricotta (page 37)
1 (24-ounce) jar dairy-free pasta sauce

Preheat the oven to 350°F.

In a medium pot, cook the shells according to package directions. Drain well.

Meanwhile, line a colander with several paper towels and press the spinach down, removing as much water as possible. In a bowl, combine the spinach and cashew ricotta and stir to combine.

When the shells are done, stuff them with the filling. Spread ½ cup of pasta sauce on the bottom of a 7-by-11-inch baking dish. Add the stuffed shells, then top with the rest of the pasta sauce, making sure the sauce coats all the shells.

Bake for 25 to 30 minutes, or until everything is heated through.

*Make it easier:* Use a store-bought dairy-free ricotta. Just mix a handful of basil and oregano into the filling for the Italian flavors.

---

**Per Serving:** Calories: 498; Total fat: 23g; Carbohydrates: 59g; Cholesterol: 0mg; Fiber: 6.5g; Protein: 19g; Sugar: 17g

# SLOW COOKER IRISH STEW

**Serves 6**

**Prep time: 20 minutes / Cook time: 4 or 8 hours**

*Egg-Free, Nut-Free, Soy-Free, Vegan*

This Irish stew is perfect for a busy winter day. Just toss the ingredients in the slow cooker in the morning, and by evening you'll have a hearty, comforting meal. Traditional Irish stews contain beef or lamb; this vegan version uses lentils instead. (Feel free to make it with meat if you'd like.) The stout beer adds an interesting depth of flavor, offering hints of bitter chocolate, coffee, and maltiness—just make sure the one you choose is dairy-free.

1 pound potatoes, peeled and cut into 1-inch chunks
1 yellow onion, chopped
2 celery stalks, chopped
1½ cups sliced carrots
1½ cups sliced mushrooms
¾ cup red lentils
2 tablespoons tomato paste
3 cups vegetable broth
1½ cups stout beer (or other dark beer)
½ teaspoon salt

Put all the ingredients in a slow cooker and mix to combine. Cook for 4 hours on high or 8 hours on low. Store any leftovers in the refrigerator for up to 4 days.

*Make it easier:* If your mornings are hectic, save time by chopping all the vegetables except the potatoes the night before. Potatoes start to brown once chopped, so save those for the morning.

---

**Per Serving:** Calories: 201; Total fat: 1g; Carbohydrates: 37g; Cholesterol: 0mg; Fiber: 6g; Protein: 9g; Sugar: 5g

# CHICKPEA STEW WITH GRITS

**Serves 6**

**Prep time: 10 minutes / Cook time: 20 minutes**

Grits aren't just for breakfast; they also make a delicious starchy alternative to pasta, rice, or quinoa for dinnertime meals. The creaminess of the grits pairs perfectly with the rich, vibrant tomato and coconut flavors in this chickpea stew. This is winter comfort food at its best, but don't let that stop you from enjoying it all year round.

- 1 tablespoon olive oil
- ½ medium red onion, diced
- 2 teaspoons minced garlic
- 2 (15.5-ounce) cans chickpeas, rinsed and drained
- ½ teaspoon chili powder
- ½ teaspoon ground cumin
- ½ teaspoon ground coriander
- ½ teaspoon paprika
- 1 (14.5-ounce) can diced tomatoes, undrained
- 1 (8-ounce) can tomato sauce
- 1 tablespoon coconut aminos or soy sauce
- 1 cup full-fat coconut milk
- 1½ cups quick grits

In a large pot, heat the oil over medium heat. Add the onion and cook, stirring occasionally, for 4 to 5 minutes, or until it starts to get tender. Add the garlic and cook, stirring, for another minute.

Add the chickpeas, chili powder, cumin, coriander, and paprika. Stir everything together, then add the diced tomatoes with their juices, tomato sauce, coconut aminos, and coconut milk. Reduce the heat to low and let simmer for 10 minutes, stirring occasionally.

Meanwhile, prepare the grits according to package directions.

Serve the grits topped with the chickpea stew. Store leftovers in the refrigerator for up to 4 days.

*Protein swap:* You can swap the chickpeas out for lentils. Just add precooked or canned lentils to the stew a few minutes before it's done simmering.

---

**Per Serving:** Calories: 370; Total fat: 13g; Carbohydrates: 55g; Cholesterol: 0mg; Fiber: 8.5g; Protein: 11g; Sugar: 6.5g

# VEGAN BEAN CHILI

**Serves 4**
**Prep time: 20 minutes / Cook time: 20 minutes**

*Egg-Free, Gluten-Free, Soy-Free, Vegan*

When those cold winter winds start howling, there's nothing more comforting than a bowl of chili. This simple vegan version is made with inexpensive pantry staples. By making your own chili seasoning mix, you'll be surprised at how much flavor you can add. Don't be put off by the cocoa powder; it doesn't make anything taste like chocolate. The rich bitterness helps cut the slight sweetness of the tomatoes.

**For the chili seasoning mix**

1½ tablespoons chili powder
1 tablespoon cornmeal
½ tablespoon ground cumin
½ tablespoon unsweetened cocoa powder
½ tablespoon paprika
½ teaspoon ground coriander
¼ teaspoon salt
¼ teaspoon freshly ground black pepper
3 tablespoons hot water

**For the chili**

1 tablespoon olive oil
1 small onion, chopped
1 bell pepper, chopped
3 jalapeño peppers, minced
2 (14.5-ounce) cans fire-roasted diced tomatoes, undrained
1 cup vegetable broth
1 (15.5-ounce) can pinto beans, rinsed and drained
1 (15.5-ounce) can black beans, rinsed and drained
Half a 15-ounce can corn kernels, drained
Cashew Sour Cream (optional, page 38)

1. **To make the chili seasoning mix:** In a small bowl, combine all the ingredients and stir well.
2. **To make the chili:** In a large pot, heat the oil over medium heat. Add the onion, bell pepper, and jalapeños and sauté for 6 to 8 minutes, or until the vegetables start to get tender. Add the chili seasoning mix and cook for another minute, stirring often.
3. Pour the canned tomatoes with their juices, the broth, beans, and corn into the pot. Simmer for 10 minutes, then serve. Top with cashew sour cream (if using). Store leftovers in the refrigerator for up to 4 days.

*Make it easier:* To save time, purchase a premade seasoning packet. Just check to ensure that it's dairy-free.

---

**Per Serving:** Calories: 292; Total fat: 5g; Carbohydrates: 50g; Cholesterol: 0mg; Fiber: 15g; Protein: 14g; Sugar: 9.5g

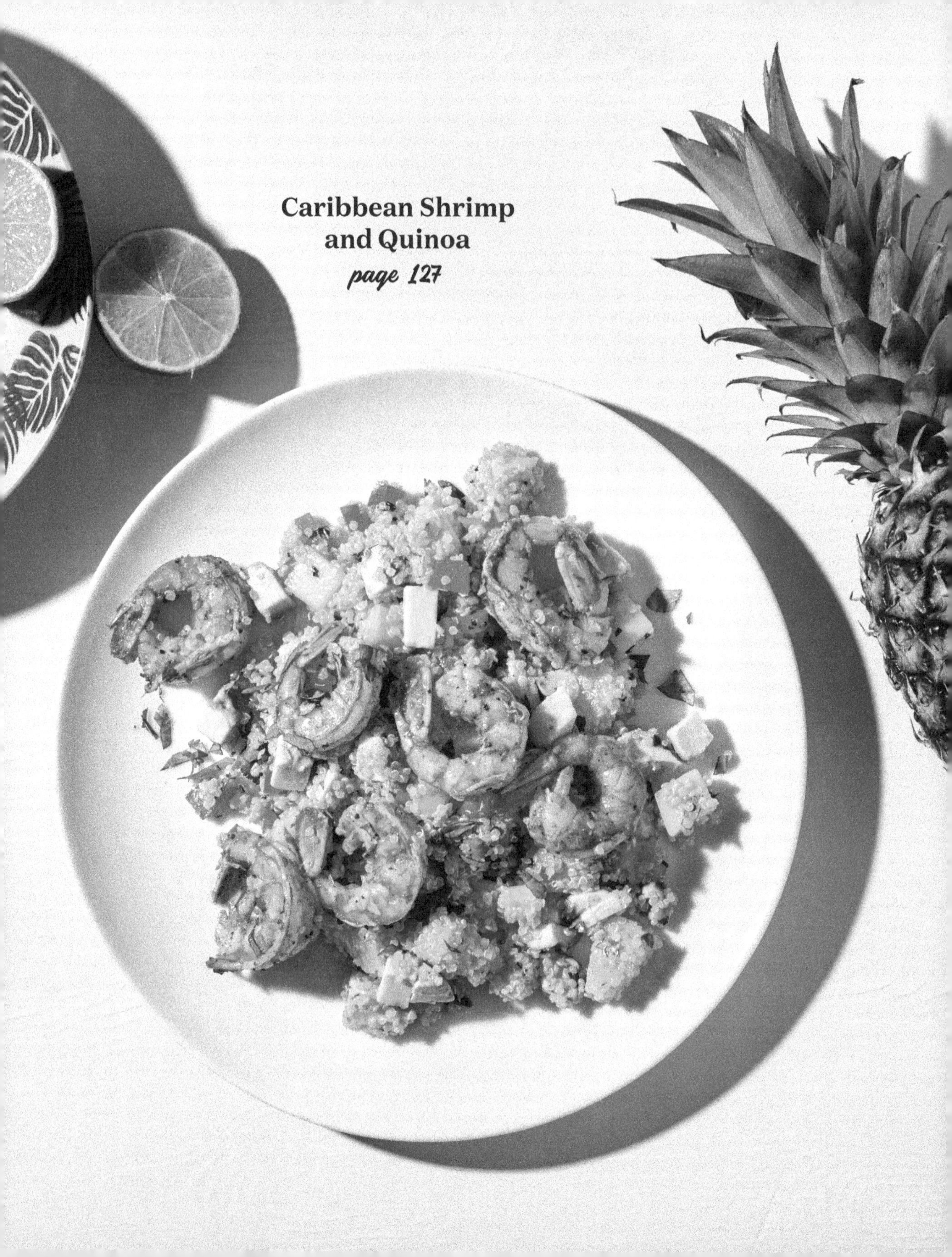

## Caribbean Shrimp and Quinoa

*page 127*

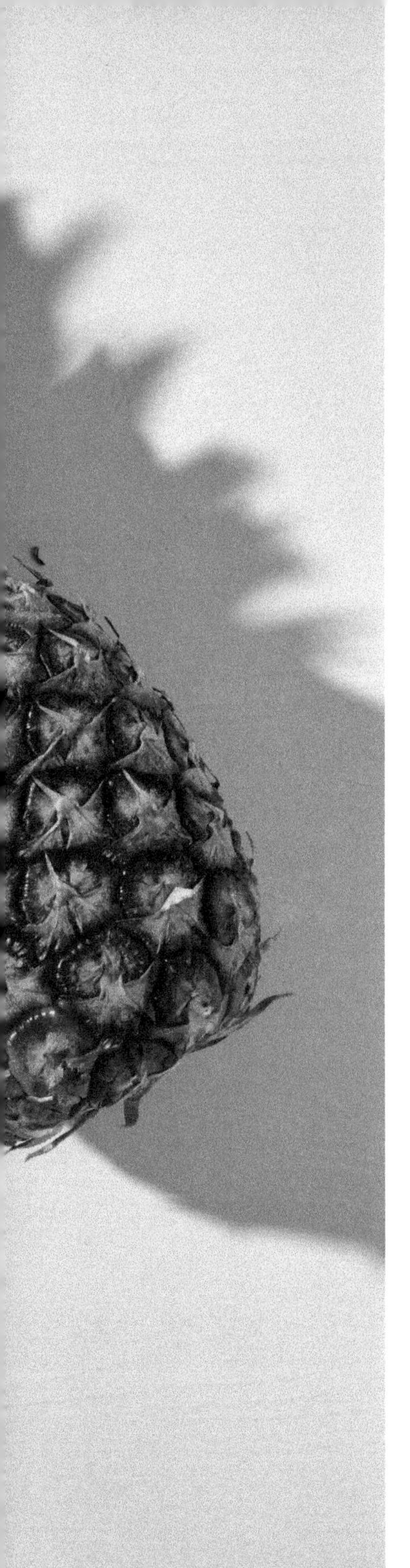

Eight

# Fish and Shellfish

# CURRIED TUNA SALAD PITA POCKET

**Makes 1 sandwich**
**Prep time: 10 minutes**

I love to keep pouches of tuna on hand for simple meal ideas. Here, tuna salad gets a boost from aromatic curry powder, bitter red onion, and sweet golden raisins. Tucked together in a whole-wheat pita pocket with fresh spinach, this easy, balanced meal satisfies and delivers omega-3 fatty acids, essential to cognitive and heart health.

1 (3-ounce) pouch tuna in water or olive oil, drained
1½ tablespoons mayonnaise
½ teaspoon curry powder
2 teaspoons chopped fresh cilantro
2 teaspoons minced red onion
1 tablespoon golden raisins
1 medium (2-ounce) whole-wheat pita bread (check to ensure dairy-free)
½ cup baby spinach

In a small bowl, combine the tuna, mayonnaise, curry powder, cilantro, onion, and raisins. Stir well.

Cut the pita crosswise in half and stuff each side with spinach, then add the curried tuna salad.

*Mix it up:* Try tossing the tuna with avocado, chopped pita bread, celery, chickpeas, lemon juice, and olive oil for an easy meal. Or use it as the protein in a quick Caesar salad.

---

**Per Serving:** Calories: 421; Total fat: 20g; Carbohydrates: 42g; Cholesterol: 29mg; Fiber: 4g; Protein: 19g; Sugar: 7.5g

# TUNA "SUSHI" BOWLS

**Serves 4**
**Prep time: 15 minutes / Cook time: 20 minutes**

*Nut-Free*

If you're a sushi fan, imagine this dish as a deconstructed California roll, but with tuna rather than imitation crab. (Though if you have crab on hand, feel free to use that!) Though regular sushi requires short-grain rice to achieve the right texture for the roll, in this deconstructed bowl, you can use any white rice you have. You can even substitute cauliflower rice for the rice if you want to boost the veggie content of the dish.

1½ cups white rice (if using instant, use 2 cups rice)
2 tablespoons rice vinegar
1 tablespoon sugar
¼ teaspoon salt
2 (5-ounce) cans water-packed albacore tuna, drained
1 cucumber, peeled and chopped
1 large avocado, chopped
2 teaspoons sesame seeds
8 roasted seaweed snack sheets, chopped into pieces
¼ cup mayonnaise
2 teaspoons sriracha sauce
2 teaspoons soy sauce (optional)

1. Cook the rice according to package directions. When done, stir in the vinegar, sugar, and salt.
2. Divide the rice among four bowls and top with the tuna, cucumber, avocado, sesame seeds, and seaweed.
3. In a small bowl, combine the mayonnaise and sriracha, then add about 1 tablespoon to each sushi bowl. Drizzle a little soy sauce over each bowl, if desired.

*Ingredient tip:* Seaweed snack sheets are generally sold in 0.35-ounce packages in the international aisle at the grocery store, or occasionally in the snack aisle with chips. In addition to using them in this dish, you can eat them as is to satisfy your salty snack cravings. If you can't find them, just leave them out of this recipe and add an extra dollop of soy sauce instead for that pop of saltiness.

---

**Per Serving:** Calories: 510; Total fat: 19g; Carbohydrates: 64g; Cholesterol: 40mg; Fiber: 4g; Protein: 22g; Sugar: 4.5g

# COCONUT CITRUS POACHED SALMON

**Serves 4**
**Prep time: 10 minutes / Cook time: 25 minutes**

This recipe was the brainchild of one of my former interns, Vee. She came up with an idea for poached salmon, and together we refined it into this tasty dish. Creamy coconut, fresh citrus, and aromatic lemongrass infuse this sauce with amazing flavor that tastes wonderful coating the tender, flaky salmon. Serve this over rice or quinoa, which will soak up every last bit of the sauce, and enjoy some sautéed greens on the side to balance out the meal.

2 fresh lemongrass stalks
1 teaspoon grated lime zest
Juice of 1 lime
2 tablespoons freshly squeezed orange juice (from about ½ orange), plus grated zest for garnish
1 cup canned full-fat coconut milk
1 (1-inch) piece fresh ginger, peeled and halved
1¼ to 1½ pounds skin-on salmon fillet (either one large fillet or several smaller pieces)
Cilantro, for garnish

Remove the tough outer leaves and the bottom woody bulb of the lemongrass. Slice a 4-inch piece from the bottom half of each stalk (discard the rest). Use the flat part of a knife to "crush" these 4-inch pieces and release the aromatic oils inside.

In a medium skillet, combine the lemongrass pieces, the lime zest, lime juice, orange juice, coconut milk, and ginger. Bring to a boil over medium heat, then reduce the heat to low and simmer for 5 minutes.

Set the salmon in the skillet, skin-side down, spooning some of the sauce over the fish. Cover and cook for 10 to 20 minutes (shorter for small fillets, longer for large fillets), occasionally spooning some sauce over the fish, until the salmon easily flakes, indicating it is cooked through.

4. Discard the lemongrass and ginger. Garnish the salmon with fresh cilantro and orange zest. Serve immediately. Store leftovers in the refrigerator for up to 3 days.

*Ingredient tip:* Lemongrass is an herb that has a strong lemon flavor and looks almost like large green onions. Look for stalks that are firm, fragrant, and green toward the top, avoiding any that are brown or dried out. Although there is such a thing as prepared lemongrass paste, the most common brand in the produce department actually contains milk as an ingredient. Skip over the processed options unless you can find a safe variety. If you can't find lemongrass, simply substitute 1 teaspoon grated lemon zest in this recipe.

---

**Per Serving:** Calories: 336; Total fat: 22g; Carbohydrates: 2g; Cholesterol: 86mg; Fiber: 0.5g; Protein: 32g; Sugar: 0g

# SHEET PAN SALMON AND VEGGIES

**Serves 4**
**Prep time: 15 minutes / Cook time: 20 minutes**

*Egg-Free, Gluten-Free, Nut-Free, Soy-Free*

Salmon is one of the most nutritious ingredients you can include in your diet, and this recipe features one of the easiest ways to cook it–just toss your ingredients on a pan and let the oven bake 'em to perfection. If you choose several smaller fillets instead of one large, you may need to shave a few minutes off the cooking time.

1 large lemon
1 (1½-pound) salmon fillet
2 cups trimmed and halved green beans
2 medium zucchini, peeled and cut into ½-inch-thick rounds
2 tablespoons olive oil
½ teaspoon salt
⅛ teaspoon freshly ground black pepper

Preheat the oven to 425°F.

Cut half of the lemon into thin slices and squeeze the juice from the other half into a small bowl.

Place the salmon on a baking sheet and surround with the green beans and zucchini. Drizzle everything with the oil and sprinkle with the salt and pepper, gently tossing the vegetables to evenly coat. Place the lemon slices on top of the salmon and drizzle the lemon juice over the vegetables.

Bake for 20 to 25 minutes, or until the fish flakes easily with a fork and the vegetables are tender.

*Protein swap:* Make this sheet pan meal with any other fish of your choice or even chicken breast. Medium chicken breasts will generally cook through in the time directed in this recipe; just ensure they reach 165°F. If using another fish in this recipe, keep in mind that thin fillets of white fish will cook much more quickly, so if needed, put the vegetables in first for 10 minutes and then add the fish in the last 10 to 15 minutes of baking.

---

**Per Serving:** Calories: 367; Total fat: 20g; Carbohydrates: 6g; Cholesterol: 108mg; Fiber: 2g; Protein: 41g; Sugar: 4g

# FISH TACOS

**Makes 8 tacos**
**Prep time: 10 minutes / Cook time: 15 minutes**

*Gluten-Free, Nut-Free*

Fish tacos are one of my favorite summertime dinners. They're light and flavorful, and I can always count on our local fish market to have a good piece of fresh white fish on hand. However, you can also make these with frozen fish instead of fresh—just allow time for the fish to thaw overnight in the refrigerator. If you forgot to move it to the fridge the night before, place the fish in a sealed bag, then submerge it in a bowl of cool water for an hour or so.

2 cups shredded cabbage or coleslaw mix
¼ cup mayonnaise
1 canned chipotle pepper in adobo sauce, finely chopped (see Ingredient tip)
Juice of 1 lime
½ teaspoon chili powder
½ teaspoon paprika
½ teaspoon ground cumin
¼ teaspoon salt
⅛ teaspoon freshly ground black pepper
1 (1¼-pound) cod fillet, cut into 4 pieces
2 tablespoons olive oil
8 corn tortillas
1 avocado, chopped
Cilantro, for garnish (optional)
Lime wedges, for serving (optional)

1. In a large bowl, mix together the cabbage, mayonnaise, chipotle pepper, and lime juice. Set aside.
2. In a small bowl, combine the chili powder, paprika, cumin, salt, and pepper. Rub the spice mix over the cod fillets.
3. In a large skillet, heat the oil over medium heat. Once hot, place the cod fillets in the pan and cook for 3 to 5 minutes per side, until the fish is cooked through and flaky.
4. Warm the corn tortillas by placing them, one at a time, over the direct flame of a gas stove or in a hot skillet. When they get a little charred on the bottom (15 to 60 seconds, depending on which method you're using), flip them with tongs to warm the other side.
5. Place half of each piece of fish on a corn tortilla, topping with a scoop of the cabbage mixture, chopped avocado, and a little cilantro to garnish (if using). If desired, serve with lime wedges for squeezing over the tacos.

*Ingredient tip:* Chipotle peppers in adobo sauce are sold in a can in the Mexican food aisle. You need just one pepper from the can for this recipe, so freeze the rest for future use in other smoky dishes, like Southwestern Turkey Burgers (page 136).

*Protein swap:* Any mild white fish works well in this dish. Mahi-mahi, halibut, grouper, snapper, or tilapia are all good choices.

---

**Per Serving (2 tacos):** Calories: 433; Total fat: 25g; Carbohydrates: 27g; Cholesterol: 60mg; Fiber: 5.5g; Protein: 26g; Sugar: 1g

# CIOPPINO

**Serves 4**
**Prep time: 15 minutes / Cook time: 40 minutes**

*Egg-Free, Gluten-Free, Nut-Free, Soy-Free*

Cioppino sounds fancy, but it's really just a catch-all fisherman's stew. It originated in San Francisco, steeped in Italian-American culture as an offshoot of Italian *zuppa di pesce*, and can be made with any kind of fish and shellfish. Be sure to serve this cioppino alongside fresh-baked crusty bread (gluten-free if needed). Dipping the bread in the flavorful broth is by far my favorite part of this meal!

- 1 tablespoon olive oil
- 1 bell pepper, chopped
- 1 onion, chopped
- 3 cloves garlic, minced
- ½ teaspoon salt
- ¼ teaspoon crushed red pepper
- 1 cup red wine
- 2 tablespoons tomato paste
- 1 (28-ounce) can diced tomatoes
- 1 (14.5-ounce) can diced tomatoes
- 3 cups chicken broth
- 1 bay leaf
- 1½ pounds fresh mussels (see Ingredient tip)
- 1 pound cod fillet (or other white fish), cut into a few smaller pieces

1. In a large pot, heat the olive oil over medium heat. Add the pepper and onion, and cook, stirring occasionally, for 5 to 7 minutes, or until the vegetables start to get tender. Add the garlic and cook, stirring, for 1 minute. Season the vegetables with the salt and crushed red pepper.
2. Pour the red wine into the pot. Increase heat to high and cook for 2 minutes. Add the tomato paste, both cans of diced tomatoes with their juices, the chicken broth, and bay leaf. Bring to a boil, then reduce heat to medium-low and simmer uncovered for 20 minutes.
3. Add the mussels to the pot and cook for 5 minutes. Add the cod and cook for another 5 to 7 minutes, until the mussels have opened and the cod is flaky and cooked through. Discard any mussels that did not open.
4. Serve immediately. Store leftovers in the refrigerator for up to 3 days.

*Ingredient tip:* Clean the mussels by placing them in a colander under running water, and scrubbing any debris on the shells. Discard any that are already open or that have broken shells. If they have "beards," a thread-like component that looks a bit like seaweed, just grab the beard with your thumb and forefinger and pull backward toward the hinged edge of the mussel to remove it.

---

**Per Serving:** Calories: 433; Total fat: 8.5g; Carbohydrates: 31g; Cholesterol: 100mg; Fiber: 6.5g; Protein: 45g; Sugar: 11g

# SEARED SCALLOPS WITH MASHED CAULIFLOWER

**Serves 4**
**Prep time: 10 minutes / Cook time: 15 minutes**

Plating white fish over white vegetables seems to be a cardinal sin in the culinary world, but I love this combination and think you will, too, so I'm going to unapologetically feature it here. The delicate, almost buttery taste of the scallops is enhanced when paired with creamy, garlicky mashed cauliflower. I recommend serving this dish alongside some easy sautéed greens if you want to make the meal more filling–and colorful. Just chop up your favorite leafy green and cook it in a skillet with olive oil for a few minutes until wilted.

**For the mashed cauliflower**

- 1 large head cauliflower, trimmed to just florets
- ¼ cup unsweetened oat milk (certified gluten-free if needed) or other dairy-free milk
- 2 tablespoons olive oil
- 2 teaspoons minced garlic
- ¼ teaspoon salt
- ¼ teaspoon freshly ground black pepper

**For the scallops**

- 2 tablespoons olive oil
- 16 large sea scallops (about 1 pound)
- ⅛ teaspoon salt
- ⅛ teaspoon freshly ground black pepper

**To make the mashed cauliflower:** Fill a medium pot halfway with water and bring to a boil over high heat. Add the cauliflower florets and boil for about 10 minutes, or until tender. Drain and leave the cauliflower in the pot.

Add the oat milk, oil, garlic, salt, and pepper and purée with an immersion blender or mash with a potato masher. Set aside.

**To make the scallops:** In a large skillet, heat the olive oil over medium-high heat. Dry the scallops and season them with the salt and pepper. When the oil is hot, place the scallops in the skillet. Let cook for about 2 minutes without moving, then flip and cook for another 2 minutes.

Add a scoop of mashed cauliflower to each plate and top each with 4 large scallops. Serve immediately.

*Ingredient tip:* The key to achieving that classic golden crust on a seared scallop comes down to two things: dry scallops and hot oil. Thoroughly dry the scallops with paper towels before searing, especially if you're using previously frozen ones, which tend to be wetter. When you place the first scallop in the pan, listen for a nice sizzle from the oil. If you don't hear that, wait for the oil to heat up more.

---

**Per Serving:** Calories: 262; Total fat: 15g; Carbohydrates: 15g; Cholesterol: 27mg; Fiber: 4.5g; Protein: 18g; Sugar: 4.5g

# STUFFING-STUFFED SOLE

**Serves 5**
**Prep time: 15 minutes / Cook time: 25 minutes**

Stuffing most commonly makes an appearance next to Thanksgiving turkey, but it's also a surprisingly excellent pairing for fish. In this case, light and flaky sole is stuffed with the seasoned bread mixture, and accentuated with a lemon topping. Serve this fish with roasted asparagus or a side salad for a delicious, balanced meal.

1 tablespoon olive oil
½ small onion, finely chopped
2 celery stalks, finely chopped
6 tablespoons vegan butter, divided
1½ cups packaged stuffing mix (check to ensure dairy-free)
½ cup chicken broth
5 sole fillets (4 to 5 ounces each)
¼ teaspoon salt
¼ teaspoon freshly ground black pepper
1 teaspoon grated lemon zest
1 tablespoon fresh lemon juice
1 teaspoon cornstarch

Preheat the oven to 400°F. Coat a 2½-quart baking dish with cooking spray.

In a medium skillet, heat the olive oil over medium heat. Add the onion and celery and cook, stirring occasionally, for 4 to 5 minutes, or until the vegetables start to get tender. Add 2 tablespoons of vegan butter and wait for it to melt, then stir in the stuffing mix and broth. Remove from the heat.

Season the sole with the salt and pepper. Add a scoop of stuffing to the center of each sole fillet, then fold the ends of the fish toward the center so they overlap. Place the fish in the baking dish with the folded ends underneath. Spread any extra stuffing around the fish in the baking dish.

Place the remaining 4 tablespoons of vegan butter in a small microwave-safe bowl and microwave for 30 seconds, until mostly melted. In another small bowl, combine the lemon zest, lemon juice, and cornstarch. Stir this into the melted butter.

Pour the lemon butter topping over the fish. Bake for about 20 minutes, or until the fish easily flakes with a fork. Serve immediately.

*Ingredient tip:* If you have leftover dry stuffing mix, save it and use it instead of the oats in the Easy Turkey Meatloaf (page 137).

*Substitution tip:* If you don't have vegan butter on hand, you can still make this dish: Use olive oil in the stuffing and mayonnaise in the topping.

---

**Per Serving:** Calories: 314; Total fat: 20g; Carbohydrates: 14g; Cholesterol: 58mg; Fiber: 1g; Protein: 18g; Sugar: 1g

# SHRIMP SCAMPI

**Serves 4**

**Prep time: 10 minutes / Cook time: 15 minutes**

*Egg-Free, Nut-Free, Soy-Free*

At the age of four, my son proclaimed himself a shrimp connoisseur; it's still by far his favorite source of protein. I can't argue with him there, because shrimp is so good, especially in this easy shrimp scampi recipe. The sauce, made with aromatic garlic and shallots along with bright citrusy lemon, is simple, yet offers plenty of flavor. We normally serve this with a simple side salad or roasted asparagus. If you're not planning to include a side, you can double up on the pasta, adding a little extra garlic, wine, and lemon juice to make enough sauce.

- 8 ounces linguine
- 2 tablespoons olive oil
- 4 tablespoons vegan butter, divided
- 1 shallot, finely chopped
- 5 cloves garlic, minced
- 1 pound shrimp, peeled and deveined
- ¼ teaspoon salt, plus more to taste
- ⅛ teaspoon freshly ground black pepper, plus more to taste
- ⅓ cup dry white wine
- 1 teaspoon grated lemon zest
- Juice of 1 lemon
- ⅛ to ¼ teaspoon red pepper flakes (optional)

1. Cook the linguine according to package directions. Drain and set aside.
2. Meanwhile, in a large skillet, heat the oil and 2 tablespoons of vegan butter over medium heat. Add the shallot and garlic and cook, stirring frequently, for 3 to 4 minutes, until fragrant.
3. Season the shrimp with the salt and black pepper. Add to the skillet and cook for 2 to 3 minutes, stirring every minute, until the shrimp turn opaque and pink. Stir in the wine, lemon zest, lemon juice, red pepper flakes (if using), and remaining 2 tablespoons of vegan butter. Cook for another minute. Add the pasta and toss everything together.
4. Serve immediately. If desired, season with more salt and black pepper. Store leftovers in the refrigerator for up to 3 days.

*Mix it up:* Instead of pasta, you can also serve shrimp scampi over rice, alongside freshly baked crusty bread, tossed with zucchini noodles, or over spaghetti squash.

---

**Per Serving:** Calories: 500; Total fat: 20g; Carbohydrates: 47g; Cholesterol: 182mg; Fiber: 2.5g; Protein: 27g; Sugar: 3g

# CARIBBEAN SHRIMP AND QUINOA

**Serves 4**
**Prep time: 15 minutes / Cook time: 20 minutes**

*Egg-Free, Gluten-Free, Nut-Free, Soy-Free*

Jerked foods originated in Jamaica, and involve rubbing meat with a dry or wet spice rub to add flavor and heat. In this case, we're departing from the traditional jerked chicken or pork and adding a spicy jerk seasoning to shrimp instead. The shellfish is definitely fiery, but the fruity Caribbean quinoa and creamy, rich avocado add balance and depth to the dish. I personally love Busha Browne's Traditional Jerk Seasoning Rub for the paste in this recipe, but there are other excellent brands on the market, too.

- 1 cup canned juice-packed pineapple chunks, plus ¼ cup pineapple juice (from the can)
- 1 mango, chopped
- 1 avocado, chopped
- ½ red bell pepper, chopped
- 1 cup quinoa
- 2 cups chicken broth
- ¼ cup chopped fresh cilantro
- Juice of 1 lime
- 2 tablespoons olive oil, divided
- 1 pound large shrimp, peeled and deveined
- 1 to 2 teaspoons jerk seasoning paste (according to spice preference)

1. In a large bowl, combine the pineapple, mango, avocado, and bell pepper. Set aside.
2. In a medium pot, combine the quinoa and chicken broth and bring to a boil over high heat. Reduce heat to medium-low, cover, and cook for about 15 minutes, or until all the liquid has absorbed and the quinoa is fluffy.
3. Stir the cilantro, lime juice, 1 tablespoon of olive oil, and the pineapple juice into the quinoa. Cover and set aside.
4. In a large skillet, heat the remaining 1 tablespoon of olive oil over medium heat. Toss the shrimp with the jerk seasoning paste and add the shrimp to the skillet. Cook for about 3 minutes, stirring every minute, until the shrimp is cooked through.
5. Add the shrimp and quinoa to the bowl with the pineapple, mango, and pepper. Toss everything and serve immediately. Store leftovers in the refrigerator for up to 3 days.

*Protein swap:* Try sautéing chicken breast or pork chops with jerk seasoning rather than the shrimp. Make the rest of the recipe as directed.

---

**Per Serving:** Calories: 511; Total fat: 17g; Carbohydrates: 64g; Cholesterol: 184mg; Fiber: 7g; Protein: 29g; Sugar: 26g

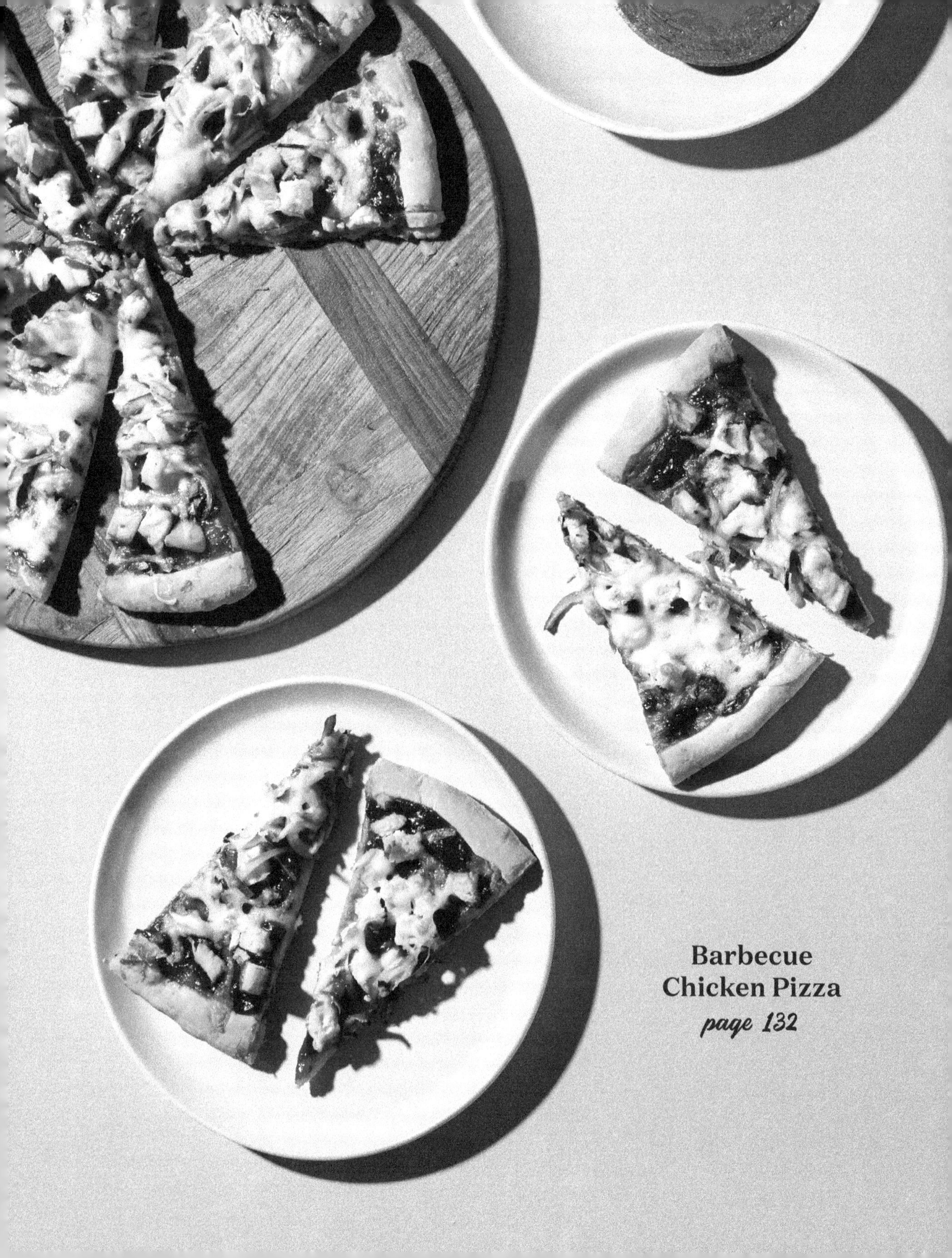

Barbecue
Chicken Pizza
*page 132*

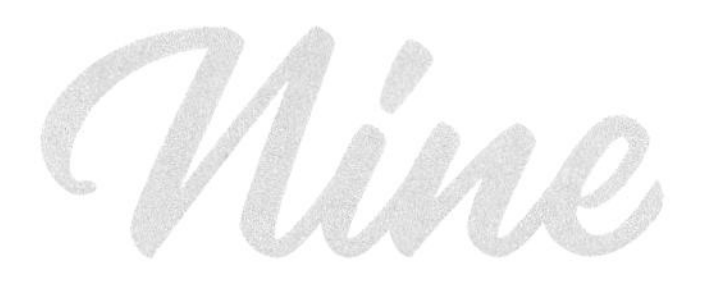


# Meat Mains

# FRIED CHICKEN

**Makes 8 pieces**
**Prep time: 10 minutes / Cook time: 40 minutes**

*Egg-Free, Nut-Free, Soy-Free*

Even as a dietitian, I'm no stranger to a plate of home-cooked fried chicken. In fact, one of my very favorite meals is chicken and waffles, which you can make using this recipe along with my Belgian Waffles (page 49), topped with pure maple syrup. The key to making great fried chicken is to get the oil to the right temperature in the pot. If the oil isn't hot enough, you'll end up with soggy skin and excess oil soaked into the chicken. If the oil is too hot, the outside will overcook before the inside fully cooks through. When you get the temperature just right, though, you'll get that golden, crispy skin and perfectly cooked interior. To test if the oil is ready, check with a thermometer, or insert a wooden spoon into the oil—when bubbles form around the spoon, it should be ready.

- 2 cups unsweetened oat milk or other dairy-free milk
- 2 tablespoons distilled white vinegar
- 1 tablespoon hot sauce
- 2 cups all-purpose flour
- 1 teaspoon paprika
- 1 teaspoon garlic powder
- 1 teaspoon salt
- ½ teaspoon freshly ground black pepper
- ½ teaspoon onion powder
- Canola oil, for frying
- 4 bone-in, skin-on chicken drumsticks (about 1½ pounds)
- 4 bone-in, skin-on chicken thighs (about 1½ pounds)

1. In a large bowl, whisk together the oat milk and vinegar. Let sit for 5 minutes, then stir in the hot sauce. In another large bowl, combine the flour, paprika, garlic powder, salt, pepper, and onion powder. Stir well.

2. Pour 3 to 4 inches of canola oil into a large pot (you want the oil to be deep enough to cover at least three-quarters of a piece of chicken). Heat the oil over medium heat for 5 to 10 minutes, until it reaches 350°F.

3. Working in two batches, dip 4 pieces of the chicken in the flour to lightly coat, shaking off any excess. Dip them in the milk mixture, then dip them back in the flour to coat again. Place the chicken in the hot oil and cook for 10 minutes, then flip if the top part of the chicken is not submerged in the oil. Cook for an additional 5 to 10 minutes, double-checking the inside of the chicken with a meat thermometer to ensure the internal temperature has reached 165°F. Remove with tongs and place on paper towels to absorb excess oil.

4. Repeat with the second batch of chicken. Cool for a few minutes before serving. Store leftovers in the refrigerator for up to 4 days.

*Cooking tip:* For perfectly reheated fried chicken, preheat the oven to 400°F and place the leftover chicken on a baking sheet to come to room temperature while the oven preheats. Bake for 15 to 20 minutes, or until the chicken is warm and the skin is crispy again.

---

**Per Serving (1 piece):** Calories: 353; Total fat: 17g; Carbohydrates: 13g; Cholesterol: 176mg; Fiber: 0.5g; Protein: 35g; Sugar: 0.5g

# BARBECUE CHICKEN PIZZA

**Serves 4**
**Prep time: 20 minutes / Cook time: 15 minutes**

Pizza can still be a Friday night indulgence when you make it yourself. The homemade crust comes together in just 15 minutes (you can also grab a store-bought dairy-free crust). Use the pizza dough as a base for any of your favorite toppings–in this case, you'll load it up with a tangy barbecue chicken mixture. Optionally, you can add dairy-free mozzarella-style shreds to this, though it tastes great without them.

**For the crust**

2 tablespoons olive oil, plus more for greasing
1 envelope active dry yeast (2¼ teaspoons)
1 teaspoon sugar
1 cup warm water (not hot)
1 teaspoon salt
2¼ to 2½ cups all-purpose flour, divided

**For the toppings**

⅔ cup barbecue sauce
1½ cups chopped cooked skinless chicken breasts or thighs
¼ cup sliced red onion
¼ cup chopped fresh cilantro
1½ cups shredded dairy-free mozzarella (optional)

**To make the crust:** Preheat the oven to 450°F. Lightly grease a baking sheet with olive oil.

In a medium bowl, combine the yeast, sugar, and warm water. Let sit for 10 minutes.

Add the 2 tablespoons olive oil, the salt, and 2 cups of flour. Continue adding flour a few tablespoons at a time, beating the dough either with a stand mixer with a dough hook or by hand, until smooth, but not tacky or dry. Let it rest for 5 minutes.

Stretch the dough and spread it on the baking sheet.

**To top the pizza:** Spread the barbecue sauce, chicken, red onion, cilantro, and dairy-free mozzarella shreds (if using) on top.

Bake for about 15 minutes, or until the crust is golden brown.

*Mix it up:* Try other tasty dairy-free toppings. Red sauce, ham or prosciutto, pineapple, and onions all make flavorful combinations. Or go classic with red sauce, dairy-free mozzarella shreds, and pepperoni.

**Per Serving:** Calories: 500; Total fat: 10g; Carbohydrates: 77g; Cholesterol: 51mg; Fiber: 2.5g; Protein: 24g; Sugar: 17g

# CHICKEN POT PIE

**Serves 6**
**Prep time: 15 minutes / Cook time: 60 minutes**

*Nut-Free, Soy-Free*

This homemade version of the winter comfort food favorite requires a little extra time in the kitchen, but it's worth it for the end result: chicken and vegetables in creamy broth all baked in a savory pie crust. Most store-bought refrigerated crusts are actually already dairy-free, helping to save a little time on this cozy classic.

2 small russet or white potatoes, peeled and cut into bite-size pieces
2 tablespoons olive oil
1 medium yellow onion, diced (about 1 cup)
1 cup diced celery
1 cup diced carrots
8 ounces baby bella (cremini) mushrooms, chopped
2 tablespoons all-purpose flour
1⅓ cups chicken broth
2 cups chopped cooked skinless chicken breasts or thighs
½ teaspoon salt
¼ teaspoon freshly ground black pepper
¼ teaspoon garlic powder
2 refrigerated dairy-free pie crusts

1. Preheat the oven to 425°F.
2. Place the potatoes in a pot and add enough water to submerge the potatoes. Bring to a boil and cook for 7 to 10 minutes, or until the potatoes are tender. Drain and set aside.
3. Meanwhile, in a large skillet, heat the oil over medium heat. Add the onion, celery, carrots, and mushrooms. Sauté for 6 to 9 minutes, or until the carrots and celery have started to get tender and the onions and mushrooms are soft and cooked through.
4. Stir the flour into the skillet and cook for about 30 seconds. Stir in the chicken broth a little at a time, letting it mix with the flour and thicken up. When all the broth is added, bring to a boil for 1 to 2 minutes to further thicken. Remove from the heat and stir in the potatoes, chopped cooked chicken, salt, pepper, and garlic powder.
5. Line a 9-inch pie plate with one of the crusts. Pour the filling mixture into the pie shell, pressing down to ensure you get as much filling in as possible without overstuffing the pie. Place the second pie crust on top, folding the sides over the bottom crust and crimping the edges with a fork. Slice a few vents in the top crust with a sharp knife.

Bake for 30 minutes uncovered, then cover with aluminum foil and bake for an additional 10 minutes. Remove from the oven and let sit for 10 minutes before serving.

*Cooking tip:* Place a sheet pan on the rack underneath the pie plate in the oven. This way, if any broth happens to bubble over, it'll drip onto the pan rather than the bottom of your oven.

---

**Per Serving:** Calories: 470; Total fat: 24g; Carbohydrates: 49g; Cholesterol: 60mg; Fiber: 2g; Protein: 20g; Sugar: 3g

# MANGO ALMOND BUTTER CHICKEN AND RICE

**Serves 4**
**Prep time: 15 minutes / Cook time: 15 minutes**

*Egg-Free, Gluten-Free*

When you're craving something unique for dinner, try this recipe. The protein-packed chicken is coated with a lovely sauce, featuring rich coconut milk, fragrant curry paste, and nutty almond butter. You'll toss this with brown rice and mango to add healthy carbs and fresh flavor for an easy, balanced meal.

- 2 cups instant brown rice
- 1 tablespoon olive oil
- 1 pound boneless, skinless chicken breasts or thighs, cut into bite-size pieces
- ½ teaspoon salt, divided
- ¼ teaspoon freshly ground black pepper
- ¼ teaspoon paprika
- 1 cup canned full-fat coconut milk
- 2 tablespoons almond butter
- 1½ tablespoons molasses
- 1 tablespoon red curry paste
- Juice of 1 lime
- 1 teaspoon yellow curry powder
- 2 mangos, chopped
- ¼ cup finely chopped red onion

1. Cook the instant brown rice according to package directions. Set aside.
2. In a large sauté pan or skillet, heat the oil over medium heat. Season the chicken with ¼ teaspoon of salt, the pepper, and paprika. Add to the pan and cook for 5 to 8 minutes, stirring a few times, until the chicken is cooked through.
3. Add the coconut milk, almond butter, molasses, curry paste, lime juice, curry powder, and remaining ¼ teaspoon of salt to the pan. Simmer for 5 minutes, stirring often.
4. Remove from the heat and stir in the rice, mangos, and red onion. Toss everything well, coating the rice with the sauce.
5. Serve immediately. Store leftovers in the refrigerator for up to 4 days.

*Protein swap:* Try turkey breast instead of chicken, or skip the meat and make this with chickpeas as the main protein source.

---

**Per Serving:** Calories: 640; Total fat: 25g; Carbohydrates: 75g; Cholesterol: 83mg; Fiber: 6.5g; Protein: 34g; Sugar: 29g

# SOUTHWESTERN TURKEY BURGERS

**Serves 4**
**Prep time: 10 minutes / Cook time: 10 minutes**

Burgers don't need cheese to be crave-worthy. These Southwestern turkey burgers are seasoned with chipotle peppers and cumin to create a flavorful, slightly smoky burger patty. Even though chipotles are spicy, the amount used here makes for very subtle heat, so they're definitely still kid-friendly. My family likes these on a bun, but I also love them tucked into a lettuce wrap or on a fried corn tortilla (tostada style).

1 pound ground turkey
2 canned chipotle peppers in adobo sauce, finely chopped
¼ cup finely chopped red onion
1 teaspoon ground cumin
¼ teaspoon salt
4 whole-wheat hamburger buns (check to ensure dairy-free)
1 avocado, mashed

In a large bowl, combine the ground turkey, chipotle peppers, onion, cumin, and salt. Mix well and form into 4 patties.

Heat a large skillet over medium heat and spritz with cooking spray. Add the burger patties and cook for 5 minutes on one side. Flip and cook for 5 to 7 minutes on the other side, until the internal temperature reaches 165°F.

Put a burger patty on each bun and top each with mashed avocado. Serve immediately. Store leftover burger patties (without the bun or avocado) in the refrigerator for up to 4 days.

*Mix it up:* Instead of avocado, try topping these burgers with spicy mayo. Mix ¼ cup mayonnaise with 2 to 3 teaspoons of the adobo sauce from the can of chipotle peppers, and spread on the burgers.

---

**Per Serving:** Calories: 360; Total fat: 15g; Carbohydrates: 26g; Cholesterol: 76mg; Fiber: 5.5g; Protein: 23g; Sugar: 3g

# EASY TURKEY MEATLOAF

**Serves 6**
**Prep time: 10 minutes / Cook time: 50 minutes**

*Egg-Free, Nut-Free, Soy-Free, Gluten-Free Option*

When my son was an infant, this turkey meatloaf was constantly on our menu because it's such an easy main dish to throw together. If I'm in a rush, I'll make a steamable bag of frozen veggies to serve with this recipe. If I have a little extra time, I like to make Creamy Mashed Potatoes (page 83) and Balsamic Honey Collard Greens (page 79) as sides.

2 pounds ground turkey
½ yellow onion, finely chopped
1 cup rolled oats (certified gluten-free if needed)
¼ teaspoon salt
¼ teaspoon garlic powder
⅛ teaspoon freshly ground black pepper
½ cup ketchup, plus ⅓ cup, divided

1. Preheat the oven to 350°F. Grease a 9-by-5-inch loaf pan.
2. In a large bowl, combine the turkey, onion, oats, salt, garlic powder, pepper, and ½ cup of ketchup. Mix well with your hands.
3. Form the meat mixture into the loaf pan. Top with the remaining ⅓ cup of ketchup. Bake for 50 to 55 minutes, or until the internal temperature reaches 165°F.

*Substitution tip:* If you don't have oats, you can substitute bread crumbs or packaged stuffing mix (check to ensure the product is dairy-free).

*Protein swap:* Feel free to use ground beef rather than ground turkey. Cook as directed.

---

**Per Serving:** Calories: 322; Total fat: 13g; Carbohydrates: 21g; Cholesterol: 104mg; Fiber: 1.5g; Protein: 32g; Sugar: 9.5g

# LEMONY TURKEY RICE SKILLET

**Serves 4**

**Prep time: 15 minutes / Cook time: 50 minutes**

*Egg-Free, Gluten-Free, Nut-Free, Soy-Free*

This one-pan meal is easy to prepare, plus satiating and nutritious. Ground turkey provides protein, and the tomatoes deliver vitamin C, potassium, and lycopene, which may help reduce cancer risk and improve heart health. The kale offers up hefty doses of beta-carotene and vitamins C and K, along with several antioxidants. Enjoy this meal knowing you're fueling your body with healthy ingredients!

½ tablespoon olive oil
1 pound ground turkey
½ cup long-grain brown rice (not instant)
½ cup wild rice
2 cups chicken broth
Grated zest and juice of 1 lemon
2 cups packed chopped kale
2 cups cherry tomatoes, halved

In a large skillet, heat the oil over medium-high heat. Add the ground turkey and cook, breaking up the meat, for 6 to 9 minutes, or until browned and cooked through.

Add the brown rice, wild rice, broth, lemon zest, and lemon juice. Bring the mixture to a boil, reduce the heat to low, cover, and simmer for 35 to 40 minutes, checking occasionally to ensure there is enough liquid for the rice, until the rice is cooked through and the liquid absorbed.

Stir in the kale and tomatoes. Increase heat to medium and cook, stirring occasionally, for about 3 minutes, until the kale is wilted. Remove from the heat and serve immediately. Store leftovers in the refrigerator for up to 4 days.

*Cooking tip:* Keep an eye on the rice as it's simmering. You may need to add more broth to the skillet if the rice has absorbed all the liquid before it's cooked through.

---

**Per Serving:** Calories: 366; Total fat: 12g; Carbohydrates: 37g; Cholesterol: 81mg; Fiber: 3.5g; Protein: 29g; Sugar: 3.5g

# APPLE-PEAR PORK CHOPS

**Serves 5**
**Prep time: 15 minutes / Cook time: 20 minutes**

*Egg-Free, Gluten-Free, Nut-Free, Soy-Free*

A good sweet and savory combo is always welcome on my dinner table. In this one, seared pork chops get a boost of sweet, fall flavors from the apples and pears. When you're cooking the topping, it will look like a lot of fruit, but you really want a heaping scoop on each chop so you have plenty with each bite of meat.

- 2 tablespoons olive oil, divided
- 5 (1-inch-thick) boneless pork loin chops (about 5 ounces each)
- ¼ teaspoon salt
- ⅛ teaspoon freshly ground black pepper
- 2 apples, peeled and sliced
- 2 pears, peeled and sliced
- 1 yellow onion, sliced

1. In a large cast iron skillet, heat 1 tablespoon of oil over medium heat. Season the pork chops with the salt and pepper. Add them to the hot skillet and cook for 4 to 5 minutes. Flip and cook for about 5 more minutes, or until the internal temperature reaches 145°F. Transfer to a plate and allow to rest.

2. Meanwhile, add the remaining 1 tablespoon of oil to the skillet and heat over medium heat. Add the apples, pears, and onion and cook for 7 to 10 minutes, stirring occasionally, until the apples and pears are tender.

3. Top the pork chops with the apple, pear, and onion mixture and serve immediately. Store leftovers in the refrigerator for up to 4 days.

***Make it easier:*** You can make this dish in the slow cooker, too. Skip the olive oil, use bone-in pork chops rather than boneless chops, cut the apples and pears into thick slices (so they don't turn to mush), and add ¼ cup of applesauce or apple juice along with the onion, salt, and pepper. Cook on high for 4 hours or low for 8 hours.

---

**Per Serving:** Calories: 388; Total fat: 21g; Carbohydrates: 21g; Cholesterol: 85mg; Fiber: 3.5g; Protein: 31g; Sugar: 14g

# SLOW COOKER PULLED PORK

**Serves 8**
**Prep time: 10 minutes / Cook time: 6 to 10 hours**

This recipe leans toward a Carolina-style pulled pork, known for its tangy vinegar sauce, rather than that made with the sweeter tomato-forward barbecue sauce. Whereas traditional Carolina 'cue is smoked low and slow over hardwood coals, we'll use the slow cooker and add a little liquid smoke, an easy way to achieve much of the same flavor profile. Once cooked, there are endless ways to use this pork—on sandwiches, nachos, omelets, salads, burritos, and more!

- 2 teaspoons salt
- 2 teaspoons paprika
- 1 teaspoon chili powder
- ½ teaspoon garlic powder
- ½ teaspoon cayenne pepper
- ¼ teaspoon ground cumin
- 4 pounds boneless pork shoulder
- 2 yellow onions, sliced
- ½ cup apple cider vinegar
- 3 tablespoons brown sugar
- 2 tablespoons ketchup
- 2 tablespoons grainy mustard
- 1 teaspoon liquid smoke

In a small bowl, mix together the salt, paprika, chili powder, garlic powder, cayenne, and cumin. Rub the mixture all over the pork shoulder.

Place the pork and onions in the slow cooker. Add the vinegar, brown sugar, ketchup, mustard, and liquid smoke.

Cook for 5 to 6 hours on high or 8 to 9 hours on low. Remove the pork and shred it on a cutting board using two forks, then return the meat to the slow cooker. Let it sit in the sauce, uncovered, on low heat for another 30 minutes.

Serve hot. Store leftovers in the refrigerator for up to 4 days. You can also freeze the pulled pork to use in later meals.

*Cooking tip:* If you try to shred the pulled pork and it feels tough, put it back in the slow cooker for another hour on high and then try again.

---

**Per Serving:** Calories: 416; Total fat: 25g; Carbohydrates: 9g; Cholesterol: 138mg; Fiber: 0.5g; Protein: 36g; Sugar: 7g

# HAM AND BLACK-EYED PEA SKILLET WITH CORN BREAD TOPPING

**Serves 4**
**Prep time: 10 minutes / Cook time: 20 minutes**

*Soy-Free, Egg-Free Option (see tip)*

Start your New Year's Day off with this recipe, and cross your fingers for a year of prosperity. Black-eyed peas have long been considered a lucky way to start the year. This superstition may be rooted in the Civil War era, when many crops were destroyed but black-eyed peas remained, offering much-needed sustenance. In the South, black-eyed peas are often cooked in dishes like Hoppin' John (a bean and rice dish) or sautéed with collard greens. I went a slightly different route, combining them with onion and ham and then topping it all off with corn bread (which happens to be another lucky New Year's food, symbolizing gold).

1 tablespoon olive oil
1 medium yellow onion, chopped
1 (15.5-ounce) can black-eyed peas, rinsed and drained
2 cups chopped ham (from a whole ham or a ham steak)
1 (8.5-ounce) box corn bread mix (check to ensure dairy-free)
⅓ cup unsweetened almond milk or other dairy-free milk
1 large egg

1. Preheat the oven to 400°F.
2. In a large cast iron skillet, heat the oil over medium heat. Add the onion and cook, stirring occasionally, for 5 minutes, or until tender.
3. Stir in the black-eyed peas and ham and cook for 1 minute. Remove from the heat.
4. In a medium bowl, mix together the corn bread mix, almond milk, and egg. Pour the mixture over the ingredients in the skillet. Use a spoon to spread it as evenly as possible over the top.
5. Transfer the skillet to the oven and bake for 13 to 17 minutes, or until the top is golden brown and a knife pulls out cleanly. Serve immediately. Store leftovers in the refrigerator for up to 4 days.

*Substitution tip:* Make this recipe egg-free by using a "flax egg." In a small bowl, combine 1 tablespoon ground flaxseed with 3 tablespoons of hot water. Let sit for 5 minutes, then use it in place of the egg in the corn bread topping.

---

**Per Serving:** Calories: 482; Total fat: 14g; Carbohydrates: 62g; Cholesterol: 92mg; Fiber: 8g; Protein: 26g; Sugar: 13g

# FRIED RICE WITH CHORIZO AND CASHEWS

**Serves 6**
**Prep time: 10 minutes / Cook time: 20 minutes**

Whenever I make a recipe that calls for rice (like the Korean Ground Beef Bowls on page 143), I like to make extra so that I can use it the next night for this dish. Leftover rice holds its texture better than fresh rice, making it ideal for fried rice. Rice that has been cooked and cooled also contains resistant starch, a type of carbohydrate that feeds the good bacteria in your gut. If you don't have any leftover rice on hand, cook some fresh for this delicious and savory dish.

4 large eggs
8 ounces dry-cured chorizo sausage (check to ensure dairy-free), sliced into ¼-inch-thick rounds
1 tablespoon olive oil
2 small heads broccoli, chopped into small florets
2 garlic cloves, minced
3 cups cooked white or brown rice
1½ tablespoons soy sauce or gluten-free tamari
1 teaspoon toasted sesame oil
3 scallions, chopped
½ cup roasted cashews

Coat a large skillet with cooking spray. Set over medium heat, add the eggs, and scramble to your preferred doneness, then set aside on a plate.

Wipe out the skillet, then coat again with cooking spray. Set over medium heat, add the chorizo, and cook for 5 to 7 minutes, or until the edges are browned. Remove with a slotted spoon and set aside.

In the same skillet, heat the oil over medium heat. Add the broccoli and cook, stirring occasionally, for 4 to 5 minutes, or until crisp-tender. Add the garlic and cook, stirring, for 1 minute.

Add the rice, soy sauce, and sesame oil and cook for about 2 minutes, until the soy sauce is absorbed. Stir in the scrambled eggs, cooked chorizo, scallions, and cashews.

Serve immediately. Store in the fridge for up to 4 days.

*Protein swap:* Instead of chorizo, try this dish with steak, chicken, or ground turkey. Chorizo is already seasoned, so you may need to add spices to compensate if you choose another meat—try a little salt, pepper, paprika, and a smidge of sriracha.

---

**Per Serving:** Calories: 432; Total fat: 26g; Carbohydrates: 30g; Cholesterol: 157mg; Fiber: 2g; Protein: 19g; Sugar: 2g

# KOREAN GROUND BEEF BOWLS

**Serves 4**
**Prep time: 10 minutes / Cook time: 20 minutes**

*Egg-Free, Nut-Free, Gluten-Free Option (see tip), Soy-Free Option (see tip).*

This recipe is a play on bulgogi, a Korean beef dish. The traditional version is made by marinating sirloin or rib eye in a soy sauce mixture, then grilling or sautéing the meat. This recipe uses ground beef instead. It's inexpensive, cooks quickly, and requires no marinating. Instead, you'll add the flavor elements right in the pan itself. By pairing the beef with broccoli and rice, you'll have an easy meal ready in under 30 minutes.

2 cups white or brown instant rice
1 (12-ounce) steamable bag frozen broccoli
1 pound ground beef
3 garlic cloves, minced
½ teaspoon minced fresh ginger
3 tablespoons brown sugar
¼ cup reduced-sodium soy sauce
2 or 3 scallions, thinly sliced

1. Cook the rice according to package directions. Set aside.
2. Cook the broccoli according to package directions. Set aside.
3. Meanwhile, coat a large skillet with cooking spray and heat over medium heat. Add the ground beef, garlic, and ginger to the skillet and cook, breaking up the meat every so often, for 6 to 10 minutes, or until browned. Drain any excess fat.
4. Add the brown sugar, soy sauce, and steamed broccoli to the skillet and cook for an additional 1 to 2 minutes, until all ingredients are well combined.
5. Serve the beef and broccoli mixture over the cooked rice and top with scallions.

*Substitution tip:* To make this recipe soy-free and gluten-free, substitute coconut aminos for the soy sauce. Since coconut aminos are naturally sweeter than soy sauce, cut the brown sugar to 1 tablespoon. Taste and adjust with additional brown sugar if necessary. For soy-free, also use olive oil rather than cooking spray.

*Make it easier:* Use shelf-stable pouches of precooked rice instead of the instant rice. This cuts down on dirty dishes and cooking time, as you can pop these in the microwave while your beef is cooking.

---

**Per Serving:** Calories: 472; Total fat: 13g; Carbohydrates: 59g; Cholesterol: 71mg; Fiber: 3.5g; Protein: 27g; Sugar: 12g

# SPAGHETTI AND MEATBALLS

**Serves 8**
**Prep time: 20 minutes / Cook time: 25 minutes**

*Egg-Free, Soy-Free Option*

There's nothing better than a big ol' plate of spaghetti and meatballs for Sunday dinner. This recipe is very easy to make, and cooking your meatballs from scratch ensures that they'll be dairy-free. (Unfortunately, most frozen meatballs contain milk.) Dairy-free bread crumbs can be tough to find, but there are several brands in both regular and panko-style—either will work in this recipe. If you can't find dairy-free bread crumbs, rolled oats are excellent in this recipe, too.

**For the meatballs**
1 pound ground beef
½ pound ground pork
½ pound ground veal (or another ½ pound of pork or beef)
2 teaspoons minced garlic
¾ cup dairy-free bread crumbs (soy-free if needed) or rolled oats
½ cup unsweetened almond milk or other dairy-free milk
½ teaspoon salt
¼ teaspoon freshly ground black pepper
1 teaspoon Italian seasoning

**For the spaghetti**
1 pound spaghetti
2 (24-ounce) jars dairy-free pasta sauce, divided
Dairy-Free Parmesan (optional, page 36)

**To make the meatballs:** Preheat the oven to 400°F.

In a large bowl, combine the beef, pork, veal, garlic, bread crumbs, milk, salt, pepper, and Italian seasoning. Form into 24 large meatballs, placing them on a baking sheet. Bake for about 25 minutes, or until the internal temperature reaches 165°F.

**Meanwhile, to make the spaghetti:** Cook the spaghetti according to package directions. Drain and return to the pot, tossing with 1 jar of pasta sauce.

Serve the meatballs with the spaghetti, topping with extra sauce from the additional jar as desired. Top with dairy-free Parmesan (if using).

Serve immediately. Store leftovers in the refrigerator for up to 4 days.

*Make it easier:* Double the meatball recipe and cook both batches. Freeze the extra meatballs in sauce in several freezer-safe containers. You can pull these out and quickly reheat in the microwave for an easy meal.

---

**Per Serving:** Calories: 531; Total fat: 16g; Carbohydrates: 62g; Cholesterol: 78mg; Fiber: 5.5g; Protein: 32g; Sugar: 10g

# SLOW COOKER POT ROAST

**Serves 8**
**Prep time: 15 minutes / Cook time: 8 hours**

*Egg-Free, Nut-Free*

Pot roast is ideal for a busy day–just toss the ingredients into the slow cooker in the morning, and by evening you'll have a complete hearty meal ready for your hungry family. The meat is fall-apart tender, and the vegetables soak up the seasonings in the brown gravy mix for a savory delight. The key to this recipe is finding the right gravy mix. Most mixes contain dairy, but a few are dairy-free. Simply Organic is probably the most easily accessible brand, but any dairy-free brand will work.

1½ pounds potatoes, peeled and cut into 1-inch cubes
1 pound carrots, peeled and chopped
1 (3- to 3½-pound) chuck roast
2 (1-ounce) packets dairy-free brown gravy mix
¾ cup water

1. Place half the potatoes and carrots in the slow cooker, then add the chuck roast. Add the rest of the carrots and potatoes around the pot roast. Sprinkle both packets of brown gravy mix over the top, then pour the water over everything. Cook on low for 8 hours.
2. Serve hot. Store any leftovers in the refrigerator for up to 4 days. The carrots and potatoes will not freeze well, but the pot roast will. Store in an airtight container in the freezer for up to 2 months.

*Mix it up:* Instead of beef, try using chicken thighs. Place 5 or 6 chicken thighs with the vegetables in the slow cooker, but instead of brown gravy mix, use this blend to season: ½ teaspoon salt, ¼ teaspoon freshly ground black pepper, ⅓ cup honey, ¼ cup ketchup, 2 tablespoons apple cider vinegar, and 2 teaspoons minced garlic.

---

**Per Serving:** Calories: 498; Total fat: 25g; Carbohydrates: 25g; Cholesterol: 152mg; Fiber: 3g; Protein: 40g; Sugar: 5.5g

# CURRY-SEASONED CABBAGE AND STEAK

**Serves 4**

**Prep time: 15 minutes / Cook time: 25 minutes**

*Egg-Free, Gluten-Free, Nut-Free, Soy-Free*

Cabbage is often underutilized outside of St. Patrick's Day, but it's actually quite versatile to cook with year-round. You can stuff it with meat and rice, shred it for tacos (like Fish Tacos, page 119), or sauté it, as in this recipe. Combining steak with curry-seasoned cabbage, carrots, and onions makes for a veggie-packed one-pan dinner. If you have leftover steak from another night's dinner, this is also a great way to repurpose that meat—just skip the first step in the recipe and proceed with the rest as directed.

2 tablespoons olive oil, divided
1 pound top sirloin steak
¾ teaspoon salt, divided
1 yellow onion, sliced
1½ cups grated carrots
1 medium head green cabbage, cored and chopped
1 teaspoon yellow curry powder
1 teaspoon ground coriander
½ teaspoon ground cumin
½ teaspoon garlic powder
¼ teaspoon cayenne pepper
½ cup chicken broth
⅓ cup chopped fresh cilantro

In a cast iron skillet, heat 1 tablespoon of oil over medium heat. Season the steak with ¼ teaspoon of salt, place in the pan, and cook for 5 minutes on one side. Flip and cook for an additional 3 to 5 minutes, depending on thickness, to medium-rare. Transfer to a plate and cover with aluminum foil. Let rest for 10 minutes.

Meanwhile, heat the remaining 1 tablespoon of oil in the same skillet over medium heat. Add the onion and carrots and sauté for about 5 minutes, or until tender.

Reduce the heat to medium-low. Stir in the cabbage, curry powder, coriander, cumin, garlic powder, cayenne, remaining ½ teaspoon of salt, and the chicken broth. Cook uncovered for 10 minutes, stirring every few minutes.

4. Cut the steak into bite-size pieces and mix into the cabbage. Stir in the cilantro. Serve immediately. Store leftovers in the refrigerator for up to 4 days.

*Protein swap:* Instead of beef, try chicken in this recipe. Cut the chicken into bite-size pieces, then sauté it in the skillet with olive oil for 6 to 9 minutes, or until cooked through. Set it aside while you prepare the vegetables and mix it back into the dish at the end.

---

**Per Serving:** Calories: 313; Total fat: 12g; Carbohydrates: 22g; Cholesterol: 79mg; Fiber: 8g; Protein: 30g; Sugar: 13g

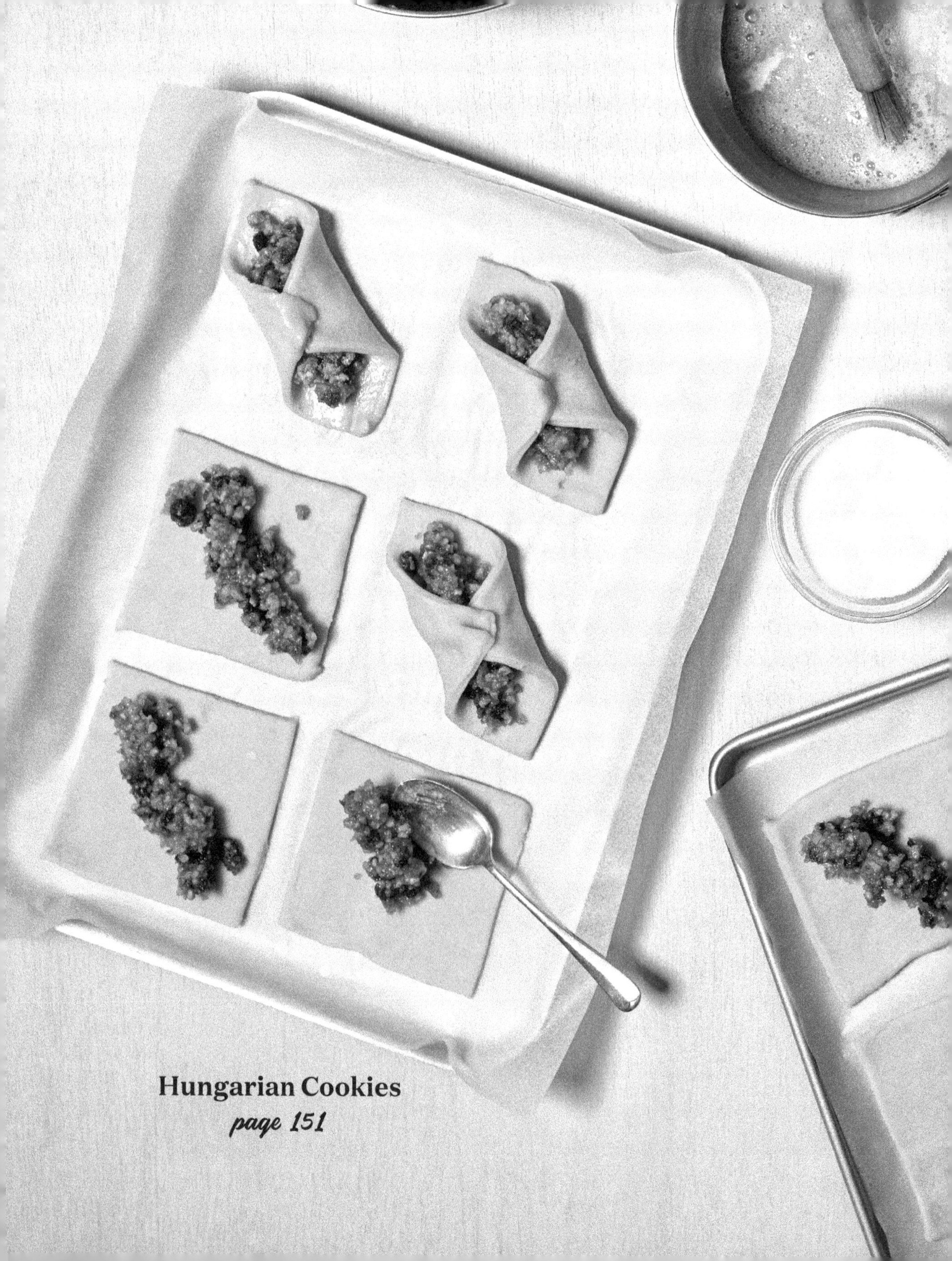

Hungarian Cookies
page 151

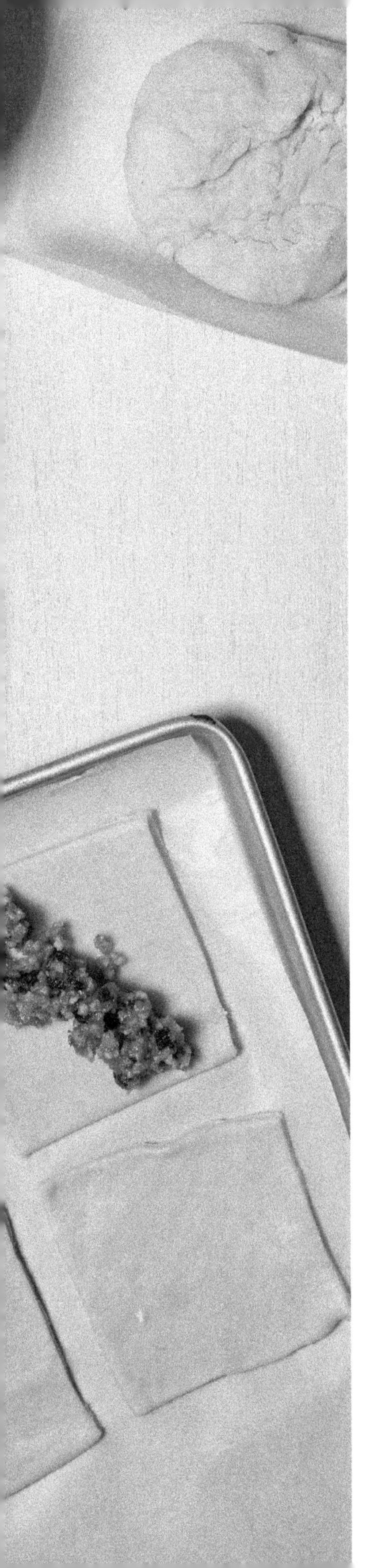

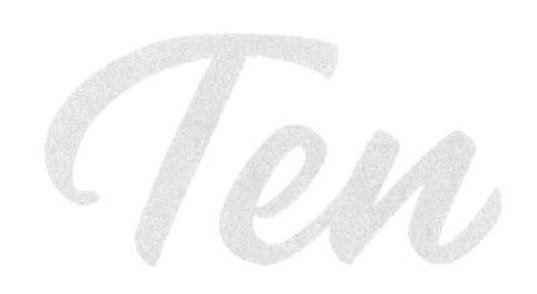

# Desserts

# FROSTED SUGAR COOKIE BARS

**Makes 9 bars**
**Prep time: 20 minutes / Cook time: 15 minutes**

*Nut-Free, Soy-Free, Vegetarian*

For birthday celebrations, think beyond cake and try these frosted sugar cookie bars instead. With a soft, chewy bar as the base and creamy vanilla frosting, these treats will make anyone smile on their special day. Quick tip: Let the cookie bars cool completely before adding the frosting. Dairy-free frosting will melt if it's put on warm cookies or cakes.

**For the sugar cookie bars**

⅓ cup vegan butter (recommended) or coconut oil
⅔ cup granulated sugar
1 large egg
1 teaspoon vanilla extract
1½ cups all-purpose flour
½ teaspoon baking powder
¼ teaspoon salt

**For the frosting**

⅓ cup vegan butter
1⅓ cups powdered sugar
1 tablespoon unsweetened oat milk or other dairy-free milk
½ teaspoon vanilla extract

**To make the sugar cookie bars:** Preheat the oven to 375°F. Grease an 8-by-8-inch baking dish.

In a large bowl, combine the butter and granulated sugar. Using a stand mixer or hand mixer, beat until fluffy. Add the egg and vanilla and beat until combined.

Add the flour, baking powder, and salt, stirring just until a dough forms.

Press the cookie dough into the bottom of the prepared baking dish. Flatten it out using your hands so it's evenly distributed. Bake for 13 to 15 minutes, or until cooked through and very lightly golden on top.

**To make the frosting:** In a bowl, combine the butter, powdered sugar, milk, and vanilla. Using a stand mixer or hand mixer, beat until creamy and fluffy.

Spread the frosting over the cooled cookie bars. Cut into 9 bars and enjoy. Store leftovers in the refrigerator for up to 4 days.

*Make it easier:* Many store-bought frostings are dairy-free, so purchase a dairy-free vanilla frosting to make this recipe even easier.

---

**Per Serving (1 bar):** Calories: 331; Total fat: 14g; Carbohydrates: 49g; Cholesterol: 21mg; Fiber: 0.5g; Protein: 3g; Sugar: 32g

# HUNGARIAN COOKIES

**Makes 16 to 20 cookies**
**Prep time: 30 minutes, plus overnight / Cook time: 15 minutes**

*Soy-Free, Vegetarian*

These cookies are inspired by my great-grandma Liz. Even into her late nineties, she'd serve three things to me and my siblings upon our visits: grilled cheese sandwiches, canned mandarin oranges, and these Hungarian cookies. She learned the recipe from her family and passed it down to my mom, who then taught me how to make them. Despite the original family recipe calling for ample butter and sour cream, I've figured out a dairy-free version that pays tribute to the classic version. They're a bit labor-intensive, but I promise you, they're worth it.

**For the dough**
½ cup coconut cream (from a can of coconut milk)
2 teaspoons fresh lemon juice
¼ cup granulated sugar
8 tablespoons vegan butter
2 egg yolks (save each white separately for the filling and topping)
½ tablespoon olive oil
2 cups all-purpose flour, plus more for dusting

**For the filling**
2 cups walnuts
½ cup golden raisins
⅓ cup granulated sugar
½ teaspoon ground cinnamon
1 egg white

**For the topping**
1 egg white
3 tablespoons powdered sugar

1. **To make the dough:** Refrigerate the can of coconut milk for 8 to 24 hours.
2. Preheat the oven to 325°F. Line a baking sheet with a silicone baking mat or parchment paper.
3. Carefully remove the can of coconut milk from the refrigerator. Open and scoop out ½ cup of the cream on top. In a small bowl, mix together the coconut cream and lemon juice and set aside.
4. In a large bowl, combine the granulated sugar, butter, egg yolks, and olive oil. Beat using a stand mixer or hand mixer. Add the coconut cream mixture, beating until fluffy. Stir in the flour until everything is just combined. Refrigerate the dough while you make the filling.
5. **To make the filling:** In a food processor, pulse the walnuts and raisins several times until the nuts are finely chopped. Pour into a bowl and stir in the granulated sugar and cinnamon.
6. In a small bowl, whisk the egg white until frothy. Pour the egg white into the walnut filling mixture, stirring well.

Remove the dough from the refrigerator and divide in half. Place the first half on a well-floured surface. Pick the dough up and flip it so it has a flour coating on both sides. Sprinkle the surface with more flour and place the dough back down again.

Roll the dough to about ⅛ inch thick. Cut it into 4-inch squares. Slide a knife underneath a square of dough and carefully place the square in your hand. Place the filling diagonally onto the square, then fold the opposite corners toward the center, pinching to join them. You'll have a log-shaped cookie with filling in the center.

Repeat this process for all the cookies, placing them on the baking sheet about 1 inch apart.

**To make the topping:** In a small bowl, whisk the egg white. Brush the egg white over the tops of the cookies. Dust with the powdered sugar.

Bake for 15 to 20 minutes, until cooked through. Let the cookies cool completely on the pan before moving them or they will crumble.

*Ingredient tip:* The dough for this is very fragile compared to regular cookie dough. Plenty of flour for rolling ensures that it does not stick, and using a knife to help you remove it from the surface is safer than attempting to pick it up with your fingers. Holding the square in your hand allows you to carefully place the filling inside and seal the edges.

*Make it easier:* Because these are labor-intensive, you may want to double the batch to make extra. You can freeze baked cookies for up to 1 month. To enjoy one (or more), let thaw to room temperature, or accelerate the process by heating in the microwave in 10-second increments.

---

**Per Serving (1 cookie):** Calories: 236; Total fat: 15g; Carbohydrates: 24g; Cholesterol: 21mg; Fiber: 1.5g; Protein: 4g; Sugar: 11g

# PINEAPPLE-COCONUT ICE POPS

**Makes 6 ice pops**
**Prep time: 10 minutes, plus 4 hours to freeze**

*Egg-Free, Gluten-Free, Nut-Free, Soy-Free, Vegan*

Who says ice pops are just for kids? These easy two- (or three-) ingredient pineapple-coconut ice pops are a hit with kids and adults alike. Enjoy their refreshing flavor after a tough day of yard work or a hot day at the beach. Just remember to account for the freezing time; make them the night before so they'll be ready to enjoy the next day.

1½ cups canned juice-packed crushed pineapple
1 cup canned full-fat coconut milk
1 tablespoon pure maple syrup (optional)

In a blender, combine the pineapple, coconut milk, and maple syrup (if using) and blend for about 20 seconds until smooth. Pour into an ice pop mold and freeze for at least 4 hours.

*Mix it up:* There are infinite flavor combinations for homemade ice pops. Start with 1½ cups of fruit (like strawberries, blueberries, or peaches) and blend with ¾ to 1 cup of liquid (like coconut milk, coconut water, oat milk, etc.) and/or dairy-free yogurt.

---

**Per Serving (1 ice pop):** Calories: 118; Total fat: 8g; Carbohydrates: 12g; Cholesterol: 0mg; Fiber: 1g; Protein: 1g; Sugar: 9.5g

# PEANUT BUTTER BANANA "NICE CREAM" PIE

**Serves 8**
**Prep time: 10 minutes, plus 6 hours to freeze**

*Egg-Free, Vegan, Gluten-Free Option (see tip), Soy-Free Option (see tip)*

This is without a doubt one of my favorite recipes in this cookbook–not only because it tastes like a mash-up between a peanut butter cup, a chocolate sandwich cookie, and banana ice cream, but also because it's so darn easy to make. You only need 6 ingredients and 10 minutes of time to whip this sweet baby up. It does need several hours to set in the freezer, but it's worth the wait.

- 1 cup peanut butter
- 2 ripe bananas, cut up
- ½ cup canned full-fat coconut milk
- ½ cup pure maple syrup
- ½ teaspoon vanilla extract
- 1 (9-inch) store-bought dairy-free chocolate cookie crust

In a large bowl, with a hand mixer or stand mixer, mix together the peanut butter, bananas, coconut milk, syrup, and vanilla. When well blended, pour into the pie crust. Freeze for at least 6 hours, then enjoy. For best quality, eat within 2 weeks.

*Substitution tip:* If you can't find a chocolate cookie crust, substitute a graham cracker pie crust instead. If you have several food allergies, check the labels to find the option that fits your needs. (There are both gluten-free and soy-free versions available.)

---

**Per Serving:** Calories: 555; Total fat: 37g; Carbohydrates: 48g; Cholesterol: 0mg; Fiber: 4.5g; Protein: 15g; Sugar: 28g

# STRAWBERRY SHORTCAKE

**Makes 9 shortcakes**
**Prep time: 30 minutes / Cook time: 15 minutes**

*Egg-Free, Nut-Free, Soy-Free, Vegan*

Strawberry shortcake has appeared in cookbooks since the mid-1800s. Shortcake doesn't refer to the stature of the dish, but to the original British meaning of the word: a crumbly texture. Normally created with copious butter in the biscuit, this dairy-free version achieves the same result using coconut oil and coconut milk. Top it off with macerated berries and Coconut Whipped Cream for a truly delicious summertime treat.

**For the berries**

2 pounds strawberries, hulled and sliced
3 tablespoons sugar

**For the shortcake biscuits**

2 cups all-purpose flour, plus more for dusting
2 teaspoons baking powder
¼ teaspoon baking soda
3 tablespoons sugar
½ teaspoon salt
4 tablespoons coconut oil
1 cup canned full-fat coconut milk

Coconut Whipped Cream (page 40) or store-bought

1. Preheat the oven to 425°F. Line a baking sheet with a silicone baking mat or parchment paper.
2. **To prepare the berries:** Combine the strawberries and sugar in a bowl, tossing to evenly coat. Place the bowl in the refrigerator for at least 30 minutes.
3. **To make the shortcake biscuits:** In a large bowl, combine the flour, baking powder, baking soda, sugar, and salt, stirring well. Use the back of a fork to cut in the coconut oil until the mixture only has small pea-size lumps left. Pour in the coconut milk and stir until combined.
4. Turn the dough out onto a lightly floured surface. Work the dough once or twice with your hands if needed so that it stays together, then flatten into a 9-inch square about 1 inch thick. Cut the square into nine 3-inch-square biscuits.
5. Place the biscuits onto the lined baking sheet and bake for about 15 minutes, or until the tops are golden brown and the biscuits cooked through.
6. Serve the warm biscuits topped with strawberries and whipped cream.

*Mix it up:* Don't hesitate to try other fruit! Raspberries, blackberries, and peaches are all solid choices for variations.

---

**Per Serving (1 shortcake):** Calories: 308; Total fat: 13g; Carbohydrates: 45g; Cholesterol: 0mg; Fiber: 3g; Protein: 4g; Sugar: 20g

# PEACH CRISP

**Serves 6**
**Prep time: 15 minutes / Cook time: 40 minutes**

Peach crisp is one of the easiest desserts to make, perfect for anyone who's not overly comfortable in the kitchen or for families baking together with their kiddos. Since ripe peaches are generally very soft, children can use a knife with a serrated plastic blade to learn cutting skills while helping you make this. The whole family will love the sweet oat topping over the warm fruit after it comes out of the oven. And of course, a scoop of dairy-free ice cream on top is always welcomed.

Canola oil, for the baking dish

**For the filling**

8 ripe peaches, peeled and sliced ½ inch thick (about 5 cups)
3 tablespoons granulated sugar
½ teaspoon vanilla extract
½ teaspoon ground cinnamon

**For the topping**

¾ cup rolled oats (certified gluten-free if needed)
⅓ cup almond flour
⅓ cup chopped pecans
⅓ cup packed brown sugar
¼ teaspoon ground cinnamon
4 tablespoons vegan butter, at room temperature

Preheat the oven to 350°F. Grease a 2½-quart baking dish with canola oil.

**To make the filling:** In a medium bowl, stir together the peaches, sugar, vanilla, and cinnamon. Pour into the baking dish.

**To make the topping:** Wipe the bowl clean, then mix together the oats, almond flour, pecans, brown sugar, cinnamon, and butter until a crumbly topping forms. Sprinkle the topping over the filling.

Bake for 40 to 45 minutes, or until the topping is golden brown and appears crisp. Serve immediately. Store leftovers in the refrigerator for up to 4 days.

*Make it easier:* Although nothing beats fresh peaches, you can also make this dish with frozen peaches. Thaw the peaches in the microwave for about 2 minutes, then use them just as you would the fresh peaches.

---

**Per Serving:** Calories: 274; Total fat: 15g; Carbohydrates: 33g; Cholesterol: 0mg; Fiber: 4g; Protein: 4g; Sugar: 23g

# PUMPKIN PIE

**Serves 8**
**Prep time: 15 minutes / Cook time: 45 minutes**

*Nut-Free, Soy-Free, Vegetarian*

Thanksgiving dinner wouldn't be complete without pumpkin pie. This recipe uses full-fat canned coconut milk instead of condensed milk or heavy cream to create a dairy-free version with all the rich flavor and silky texture you're craving. Many other milk alternatives, like almond milk, are thinner than coconut milk, so although the filling will still taste great if you sub in one of those choices, it won't have the same velvety mouthfeel.

3 large eggs
1 (15-ounce) can unsweetened pumpkin purée
1 cup canned full-fat coconut milk
¾ cup sugar
1 teaspoon vanilla extract
1 teaspoon ground cinnamon
½ teaspoon salt
¼ teaspoon ground cloves
¼ teaspoon ground ginger
1 refrigerated dairy-free pie crust

1. Preheat the oven to 425°F.
2. In a large bowl, whisk the eggs. Stir in the pumpkin purée, coconut milk, sugar, vanilla, cinnamon, salt, cloves, and ginger.
3. Line a 9-inch pie plate with the pie crust, then pour in the filling. Bake for 15 minutes, then reduce the oven temperature to 350°F and bake for an additional 30 minutes, or until the filling is just set.
4. Let sit for 30 minutes before serving. Store leftover pie in the refrigerator for up to 4 days.

*Substitution tip:* Use 1½ teaspoons of pumpkin pie spice in place of the cinnamon, cloves, and ginger.

---

**Per Serving:** Calories: 285; Total fat: 15g; Carbohydrates: 37g; Cholesterol: 75mg; Fiber: 1.5g; Protein: 4g; Sugar: 21g

# CINNAMON SUGAR BISCUIT DONUTS

**Makes 10 donuts**

**Prep time: 5 minutes / Cook time: 15 minutes**

*Egg-Free, Nut-Free, Vegan*

On Christmas morning as a child, I could look forward to two constants–presents from Santa and these cinnamon sugar "biscuit donuts" for breakfast. My mom taught me how to make this simple recipe, which I now make for my family every holiday season. Two quick tips: First, make sure the biscuits you choose are on the smaller side (not the jumbo ones). Second, double-check that they're dairy-free. Not all brands are, but many–even some labeled "buttermilk biscuits"–are dairy-free.

⅓ cup sugar
1 teaspoon ground cinnamon
Canola oil, for frying
1 (7.5-ounce) can refrigerated dairy-free biscuits (10 small biscuits)

1. In a small bowl, mix together the sugar and cinnamon. Set aside.
2. Pour 1 inch of canola oil into a sauté pan or skillet. Heat over medium heat for a few minutes, until the oil reaches 350°F (see Cooking tip).
3. Take each biscuit from the can and poke and stretch a hole in the center to form a donut shape. Working in batches so you don't crowd the pan, place the biscuits in the oil and fry for 1 to 2 minutes per side, until golden brown and cooked through.
4. Remove each donut and dip both sides in the cinnamon sugar mixture, then set aside on a paper towel to blot any excess oil. Serve immediately–these donuts don't reheat well.

*Cooking tip:* If you don't have a thermometer, test the oil by adding a small pinch of biscuit dough. If it sizzles and gets golden brown in a minute or two, the oil is ready. If it browns too quickly or starts smoking, the oil is too hot. If it doesn't sizzle and takes more than a few minutes to brown, the oil is not hot enough.

*Mix it up:* Instead of dipping these in cinnamon sugar, mix together 2 cups powdered sugar, 1 teaspoon vanilla, and a few splashes of dairy-free milk. Dip the donuts in the glaze.

---

**Per Serving (1 donut):** Calories: 129; Total fat: 7g; Carbohydrates: 16g; Cholesterol: 0mg; Fiber: 0.5g; Protein: 1g; Sugar: 8g

# CHOCOLATE CAKE WITH MARSHMALLOW BUTTERCREAM FROSTING

**Serves 16**

**Prep time: 25 minutes / Cook time: 25 minutes**

*Nut-Free, Soy-Free, Vegetarian*

There's nothing quite like a fluffy, rich piece of chocolate cake. This version is frosted with a rich marshmallow buttercream, which gives the cake a subtle s'mores-like flavor. If you want to accentuate that feature, add some crushed graham crackers in the center layer and on top. Although this recipe does have a longer list of ingredients, they're almost all baking staples that are probably already in your pantry.

**For the cake**

½ cup canola oil, plus more for greasing
⅔ cup unsweetened oat milk or other dairy-free milk
½ tablespoon distilled white vinegar
1¾ cups granulated sugar
1 teaspoon vanilla extract
3 large eggs
1¾ cups all-purpose flour
¾ cup unsweetened cocoa powder
1½ teaspoons baking powder
½ teaspoon baking soda
½ teaspoon salt
½ cup hot water

**To make the cake:** Preheat the oven to 350°F. Grease two 9-inch cake pans well with canola oil.

Combine the milk and vinegar in a glass. Set aside.

In a large bowl, mix together the ½ cup of oil, granulated sugar, and vanilla. Whisk in the eggs.

In another large bowl, combine the flour, cocoa powder, baking powder, baking soda, and salt. Pour the dry ingredients into the wet ingredients. Add the hot water and stir. Add the milk mixture and stir until everything is just combined. Pour into the prepared cake pans.

Bake for 25 to 30 minutes, or until a toothpick inserted in the center comes out clean. Let cool for 10 to 15 minutes in the pans, then place a plate on top and invert each pan to remove the cakes. If they stick to the pan, tap the bottom of the pan several times firmly until they pop out. Let the cakes cool before frosting.

**For the frosting**

1 (7.5-ounce) container marshmallow creme (such as Marshmallow Fluff)
1 cup (2 sticks) vegan butter, at room temperature
1½ cups powdered sugar
½ teaspoon vanilla extract
2 tablespoons unsweetened oat milk or other dairy-free milk

6. **Meanwhile, make the frosting:** In a large bowl, combine the marshmallow creme, butter, powdered sugar, vanilla, and milk. Use a stand mixer or hand mixer to beat until light and fluffy.

7. When the cakes are completely cool, set one layer on a cake plate. Spread with frosting and place the second layer on top. Frost the top and sides of the cake. Serve immediately. Store leftovers in the refrigerator for up to 4 days.

*Make it easier:* Many store-bought frostings are dairy-free. This cake tastes great with store-bought vanilla or coconut pecan frosting.

---

**Per Serving:** Calories: 416; Total fat: 20g; Carbohydrates: 58g; Cholesterol: 35mg; Fiber: 2g; Protein: 3g; Sugar: 42g

# NO-BAKE BROWNIE BITES

**Makes 12 large or 24 small brownie bites**
**Prep time: 15 minutes, plus 1 hour to chill**

*Egg-Free, Gluten-Free, Soy-Free, Vegan*

When you've got a chocolate craving calling your name, this will answer the call. It's so rich and indulgent, you won't believe that it's made with nutritious ingredients. Nuts in the base provide healthy fats, cocoa powder offers a dose of chocolate flavor and health-boosting flavanols, and dates naturally sweeten the raw brownies and increase the fiber content. The frosting is optional, but highly recommended.

**For the base**

1½ cups pitted dates
1½ cups pecans or walnuts
½ cup unsweetened cocoa powder
2 tablespoons cashew butter
2 tablespoons dairy-free dark chocolate chips
½ teaspoon vanilla extract
¼ teaspoon salt

**For the frosting (optional but recommended)**

4 tablespoons vegan butter
⅓ cup pure maple syrup
¾ cup unsweetened cocoa powder
2 to 3 tablespoons vanilla almond milk

**To make the base:** In a food processor, combine the dates, pecans, cocoa powder, cashew butter, chocolate chips, vanilla, and salt and process for about 60 seconds. Scrape down the sides and turn on for another 30 to 60 seconds, or until the mixture is well combined.

Pour the mixture into an 8-by-8-inch dish lined with parchment paper. Press the mixture down very firmly.

**To make the frosting:** In a bowl, combine the butter, maple syrup, cocoa powder, and 2 tablespoons of milk. Using a hand mixer or stand mixer, whisk well until it forms a fluffy frosting, adding another 1 tablespoon of milk if needed. Spread the frosting over the base mixture.

Refrigerate for at least 1 hour.

Cut into bite-size squares, leaving them in the dish until you're ready to eat. Store in the refrigerator for up to 4 days.

*Substitution tip:* If you can't find vegan butter, try chocolate ganache frosting instead: Heat 1 cup of coconut cream and whisk in 1 cup of dairy-free chocolate (chips or chopped pieces). When combined, let cool for a few minutes, then spread over the raw brownies.

---

**Per Serving (1 large bite with frosting):** Calories: 231; Total fat: 16g; Carbohydrates: 26g; Cholesterol: 0mg; Fiber: 6g; Protein: 4g; Sugar: 17g

**Per Serving (1 large bite without frosting):** Calories: 174; Total fat: 12g; Carbohydrates: 20g; Cholesterol: 0mg; Fiber: 6g; Protein: 4g; Sugar: 11g

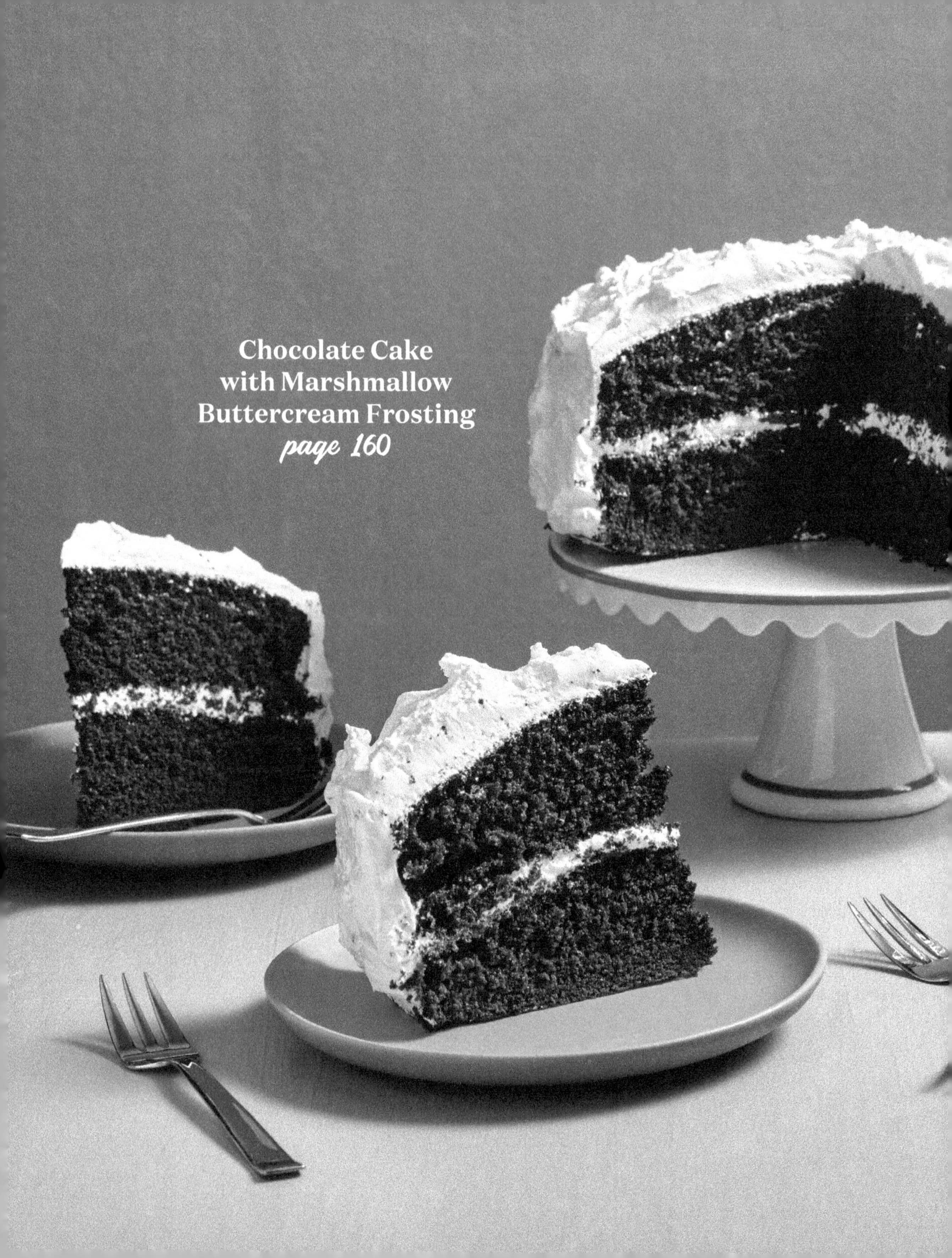
Chocolate Cake
with Marshmallow
Buttercream Frosting
page 160

# MEASUREMENT CONVERSIONS

| | US STANDARD | US STANDARD (OUNCES) | METRIC (APPROXIMATE) |
|---|---|---|---|
| VOLUME EQUIVALENTS (LIQUID) | 2 TABLESPOONS | 1 FL. OZ. | 30 ML |
| | ¼ CUP | 2 FL. OZ. | 60 ML |
| | ½ CUP | 4 FL. OZ. | 120 ML |
| | 1 CUP | 8 FL. OZ. | 240 ML |
| | 1½ CUPS | 12 FL. OZ. | 355 ML |
| | 2 CUPS OR 1 PINT | 16 FL. OZ. | 475 ML |
| | 4 CUPS OR 1 QUART | 32 FL. OZ. | 1 L |
| | 1 GALLON | 128 FL. OZ. | 4 L |
| VOLUME EQUIVALENTS (DRY) | ⅛ TEASPOON | | 0.5 ML |
| | ¼ TEASPOON | | 1 ML |
| | ½ TEASPOON | | 2 ML |
| | ¾ TEASPOON | | 4 ML |
| | 1 TEASPOON | | 5 ML |
| | 1 TABLESPOON | | 15 ML |
| | ¼ CUP | | 59 ML |
| | ⅓ CUP | | 79 ML |
| | ½ CUP | | 118 ML |
| | ⅔ CUP | | 156 ML |
| | ¾ CUP | | 177 ML |
| | 1 CUP | | 235 ML |
| | 2 CUPS OR 1 PINT | | 475 ML |
| | 3 CUPS | | 700 ML |
| | 4 CUPS OR 1 QUART | | 1 L |
| | ½ GALLON | | 2 L |
| | 1 GALLON | | 4 L |
| WEIGHT EQUIVALENTS | ½ OUNCE | | 15 G |
| | 1 OUNCE | | 30 G |
| | 2 OUNCES | | 60 G |
| | 4 OUNCES | | 115 G |
| | 8 OUNCES | | 225 G |
| | 12 OUNCES | | 340 G |
| | 16 OUNCES OR 1 POUND | | 455 G |

| | FAHRENHEIT (F) | CELSIUS (C) (APPROXIMATE) |
|---|---|---|
| OVEN TEMPERATURES | 250°F | 120°C |
| | 300°F | 150°C |
| | 325°F | 180°C |
| | 375°F | 190°C |
| | 400°F | 200°C |
| | 425°F | 220°C |
| | 450°F | 230°C |

# RECOMMENDED BRANDS

Finding store-bought substitutes for certain dairy staples can be challenging. Although all taste buds are different, here are a few of my favorite brands.

*Note: Manufacturer formulations can change at any time; always double-check the labels prior to purchasing.*

## DAIRY-FREE MILKS

365 Everyday Value Organic Coconut Milk (Whole Foods brand)

Almond Breeze

Califia

Oatly

Planet Oat

Ripple

Silk

## DAIRY-FREE CHEESE

365 Everyday Value plant-based cheddar cheese alternative, shredded (Whole Foods brand)

Chao vegan slices

Follow Your Heart cheese alternative (especially the smoked gouda)

Siete cashew queso

Violife vegan cheddar shreds

WayFare cream cheese

### YOGURT ALTERNATIVES

Dairy-Free Oui by Yoplait

Forager Project

So Delicious

Silk (soymilk and oatmilk yogurt for snacking; almond milk yogurt for making dips)

### BUTTER ALTERNATIVES

Country Crock Plant Butter (olive oil, avocado oil, or almond-oil bases)

Earth Balance

Miyoko's Creamery

### FROZEN WHIPPED TOPPINGS

So Delicious CocoWhip

Truwhip

### ICE CREAM ALTERNATIVES

Archer Farms nondairy frozen desserts (Target brand)

Ben & Jerry's nondairy frozen desserts

Cado avocado frozen desserts

Häagen-Dazs nondairy

NadaMoo dairy-free frozen desserts

So Delicious nondairy frozen desserts

## DRESSINGS

JUST Ranch

Kraft Creamy Italian Dressing

Panera at Home Caesar Dressing

Primal Kitchen Salad Dressings

## PANTRY STAPLES

Arrowhead Mills Organic Stuffing, Savory Herb

Campbell's Condensed Golden Mushroom Soup (can often be used as a substitute for cream of mushroom soup in recipes)

Otamot Pasta Sauces

Primal Kitchen No Dairy Alfredo Sauce

RAGÚ sauces: Simply™ Roasted Garlic and Simply™ Chunky Garden Vegetable

Simply Organic Brown Gravy Mix

Stove Top Stuffing Mix

## BAKING STAPLES

Annie's Cinnamon Rolls (refrigerated)

Duncan Hines Chewy Fudge Brownie Mix

Enjoy Life Chocolate Chips

Jiffy Corn Muffin Mix

Marshmallow Fluff

Pillsbury Buttermilk Biscuits (regular, *not* Grands or Flaky Layers)

Pillsbury Crescent Rolls (refrigerated)

Pillsbury Pie Crusts (refrigerated)

Simply Delicious Chocolate Chips: semi-sweet, dark, and white (Nestlé Toll House brand—note that only their Simply Delicious line is dairy-free, so double-check the packaging)

## SNACKS

ALDI Brownie Batter Dessert Hummus

Enjoy Life products (cookies, crackers, bars)

Nature's Bakery Fig Bars

Oreos

Pringles Original Flavor

Ritz Crackers

Siete Tortilla Chips

Teddy Grahams

Wheat Thins Original

# RESOURCES

The following websites and books will help on your journey to dairy-free living:

Going dairy-free:

- dairyfreeforbaby.com
- makeitdairyfree.com
- godairyfree.org

Dining out:

- allergyeats.com
- godairyfree.org/news/allergy-friendly-restaurant-chains

Cooking:

- *The 30-Minute Dairy Free Cookbook: 101 Easy and Delicious Meals for Busy People* by Silvana Nardone

# REFERENCES

Aune D, Keum N, Giovannucci E, et al. "Dietary intake and blood concentrations of anti-oxidants and the risk of cardiovascular disease, total cancer, and all-cause mortality: A systematic review and dose-response meta-analysis of prospective studies." *Am J Clin Nutr.* 2018;108(5):1069–1091. doi:10.1093/ajcn/nqy097

Connors L, O'Keefe A, Rosenfield L, Kim H. "Non-IgE-mediated food hypersensitivity." *Allergy Asthma Clin Immunol.* 2018;14(Suppl 2):56. doi:10.1186/s13223-018-0285-2

Espín J, Díaz M, Blesa B, Claver M, Hernández H, García B, Mérida M, Pinto F, Coronel R, Román R, Ribes K. "Non-IgE-mediated cow's milk allergy: Consensus document of the Spanish Society of Paediatric Gastroenterology, Hepatology, and Nutrition (SEGHNP), the Spanish Association of Paediatric Primary Care (AEPAP), the Spanish Society of Extra-hospital Paediatrics and Primary Health Care (SEPEAP), and the Spanish Society of Paediatric Clinical Immunology, Allergy, and Asthma (SEICAP)." *An Pediatr* (Barc). 2019 Mar;90(3):193.e1-193.e11. doi: 10.1016/j.anpedi.2018.11.007

Food Allergy Research and Education. Milk Allergy. Foodallergy.org. https://www.foodallergy.org/common-allergens/milk-allergy. Accessed December 6, 2019.

Huang J, Weinstein SJ, Yu K, Männistö S, Albanes D. "Serum beta carotene and overall and cause-specific mortality." *Circ Res.* 2018;123(12):1339–1349. doi:10.1161/CIRCRESAHA.118.313409

Juhl CR, Bergholdt HKM, Miller IM, Jemec GBE, Kanters JK, Ellervik C. "Dairy intake and acne vulgaris: A systematic review and meta-analysis of 78,529 children, adolescents, and young adults." *Nutrients.* 2018;10(8):1049. doi:10.3390/nu10081049

# INDEX

## D



## E



## F



## G



## H

## T



## V



## W

# ABOUT THE AUTHOR

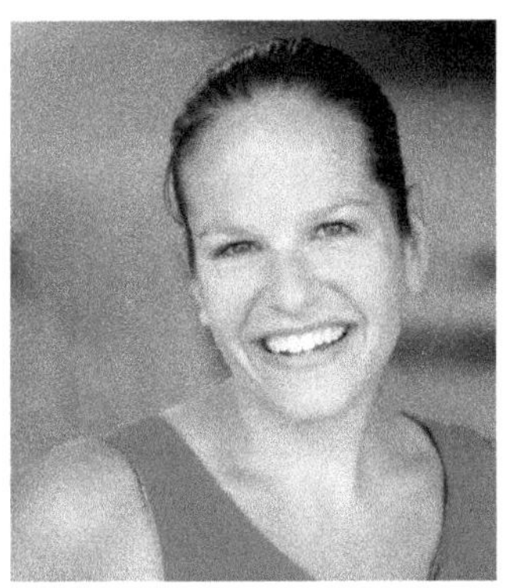

**Chrissy Carroll** is a vibrant registered dietitian and USAT Level I Triathlon coach. She currently owns several food websites, and is also a freelance writer and nutrition communications consultant.

One of Chrissy's websites, *Dairy Free for Baby*, specifically focuses on tasty dairy-free recipes and helpful nutrition tips for families with food allergies. She's especially passionate about helping this group after her own son was born with several food intolerances (which he luckily outgrew). Chrissy holds a bachelor of nutrition science from Boston University and a master of public health nutrition from the University of Massachusetts Amherst. On the personal front, she is a runner and triathlete who loves binge-watching *Top Chef*. She currently resides in central Massachusetts with her husband and son.

CPSIA information can be obtained
at www.ICGtesting.com
Printed in the USA
BVHW090553221121
622132BV00004B/8